SAME SOUL,
MANY BODIES

ALSO BY BRIAN L. WEISS, M.D.

Many Lives, Many Masters

Through Time into Healing

Only Love Is Real

Messages from the Masters

*Meditation: Achieving Inner Peace and
Tranquility in Your Life*

DR BRIAN WEISS

SAME SOUL, MANY BODIES

PIATKUS

CONTENTS

AUTHOR'S NOTE

In this book, names and other identifying information—occupations or professions, geographical facts (cities, streets), etc.—have been changed. Other than the alteration of such identifying information, the events in the sessions are reproduced as they occurred.

You will undoubtedly spot some anachronisms in the dialogue, as certain critics have in my earlier books. In *Many Lives, Many Masters,* for example, the B.C. date that Catherine mentions invalidated her story for them, but this "proof of inauthenticity" to the skeptics is fool's gold. It is easily explained by the fact that all my patients' memories are filtered through contemporary minds. They are aware of today, though their memories are from the past—and, in this book, the future.

There is one and the same soul in many bodies.

PLOTINUS

PREFACE

Recently, I've been going to a place I've rarely been before: the future.

When Catherine came to me as a psychiatric patient twenty-four years ago, she recalled with stunning accuracy her travels into past lives she had led that were as far apart as the second millennium B.C. and the middle of the twentieth century, thereby changing my life forever. Here was a woman who reported experiences and descriptions from centuries past that she could not have known in this life, and I—a Yale- and Columbia-trained psychiatrist, a *scientist*—and others were able to validate them. Nothing in my "science" could explain it. I only knew that Catherine was reporting what she had actually seen and felt.

As Catherine's therapy progressed, she brought back lessons from the Masters—incorporeal guides or spirits possessed of great wisdom—who surrounded her when she was detached from her body. This wisdom has informed my thought and governed my behavior ever since. Catherine could go so deeply into the past and had such transcendent experiences that, listening to her, I felt a sense of magic and mystery. Here were realms I never knew existed. I was exhilarated, astonished—and scared. Who would believe me? Did I believe myself? Was I mad? I felt like a little boy with a secret that, when revealed, would change the way we view life forever. Yet I sensed that no one would listen. It took me four years to gather the courage to write of Catherine's and my voyages in *Many Lives, Many Masters*. I feared I would be cast out of the psychiatric community, yet I became more and more sure that what I was writing was true.

In the intervening years my certainty has solidified, and many others, patients and therapists, have acknowledged the truth of my findings. By now I have helped more than four thousand patients by bringing them back through hypnosis to their past lives, so my sense of shock at the *fact* of reincarnation, if not the fascination of discovery, has worn off. But now the shock is back, and I am revitalized by the implications. I can now bring my patients into the future and see it with them.

Actually, I once tried to take Catherine into the future, but she talked not of her own future but of mine, seeing my death clearly. It was unsettling to say the least! "When your tasks are completed, your life will be ended," she told me, "but there's much time before then. Much time." Then she drifted into a different level, and I learned no more.

Months later I asked her if we could go into the future again. I was talking directly to the Masters then as well as to her subconscious mind, and they answered for her: *It is not allowed.* Perhaps seeing into the future would have frightened her too much. Or maybe the timing wasn't right. I was young and probably couldn't have dealt as competently with the unique dangers that progression into the future posed as I can now.

For one thing, progressing into the future is more difficult for a therapist than going into the past because the future has not yet happened. What if what a patient experiences is fantasy, not fact? How can we validate it? We can't. We know that when we go back to past lives, events have already happened and in many cases can be proven. But let's suppose a woman of childbearing age sees the world as being destroyed in twenty years. "I'm not going to bring a child into this world," she thinks. "It will die too soon." Who's to say her vision is real? That her decision was logical? She'd have to be a very mature person to understand that what she saw might be distortion, fantasy, metaphor, symbolism, the actual future, or perhaps a mixture of all of these. And what if a person foresaw his death in two years—a death caused by, say, a drunk driver? Would he panic? Never drive again? Would the vision induce anxiety attacks? No, I told myself. Don't go there. I became concerned about self-fulfilling prophecy and the unstable person. The risks of acting on delusion were too great.

Still, over the twenty-four years since Catherine was my patient, a few others have gone into the future spontaneously, often toward the end of their therapy. If I felt confident of their ability to understand that what they were witnessing might be fantasy, I encouraged them to go on. I'd say, "This is about growth and experiencing, helping you now to make proper and wise decisions. But we're going to avoid any memories (yes, memories of the future!), visions, or connections to any death scenes or serious illnesses. This is only for learning." And their minds would do that. The therapeutic value was appreciable. I found that these people were making wiser decisions and better choices. They could look at a near future fork in the road and say, "If I take this path, what will happen? Would it be better to take the other?" And sometimes their look at the future would come true.

Some people who come to me describe precognitive events: knowing what will happen before it happens. Researchers into near death experiences write about this; it's a concept that goes back to prebiblical times. Think of Cassandra who could accurately foretell the future but who was never believed.

The experience of one of my patients demonstrates the power and perils of precognition. She began having dreams of the future, and often what she dreamed came to pass. The dream that precipitated her coming to me was of her son being in a terrible car accident. It was "real," she told me. She saw it clearly and was panicked that her son would die in that way. Yet the man in the dream had white hair, and her son was a dark-haired man of twenty-five.

"Look," I said, feeling suddenly inspired, thinking of Catherine and sure that my advice was right, "I know that many of your dreams have come true, but it doesn't mean that this one will. There are spirits—whether you call them angels, guardians, guides, or God, it's all higher energy, higher consciousness around us. And they can intervene. In religious terms this is called grace, the intervention by a divine being. Pray, send light, do whatever you can in your own way."

She took my words literally and prayed, meditated, wished for, and revisualized. Still, the accident happened. Only it wasn't a fatal accident. There had been no need for her to panic. True, her son suffered head injuries, but there was no serious damage. Nevertheless, it was a traumatic event for him: When the doctors removed the bandages from his head, they saw that his hair had turned white.

Until a few months ago, on those rare occasions when I progressed my patients forward, it was usually into their own lifetimes. I did the progressions only when I thought the patient was psychologically strong enough to handle them. Often I was as unsure as they were about the meaning of the scenes they brought back.

Last spring, however, I was giving a series of lectures on a cruise ship. In such sessions I often hypnotize my listeners en masse, then lead them into an earlier life and back again to the present. Some go back in time, some fall asleep, others stay where they are, unhypnotized. This time a member of the audience— Walter, a wealthy man who is a genius in the software business— went into the future on his own. And he didn't go into his own lifetime, he jumped a millennium ahead!

He had come through dark clouds to find himself in a different world. Some of the areas, such as the Middle East and North Africa, were "off limits," perhaps because of radiation damage, perhaps because of an epidemic, but the rest of the world was beautiful. There were far fewer people inhabiting it, because of nuclear catastrophe or plague or the lowering of the fertility rate. He remained in the countryside and so could not speak about cities, but the people were content, happy, even blissful. He said he hadn't the right words to describe their state. Whatever had thinned the population had happened long before. What he saw was idyllic. He wasn't sure of the date, but he was sure that it was more than a thousand years from now.

The experience helped him emotionally. He was rich enough to fantasize about changing the world, but now he realized no one man could do that. There are too many politicians, he said, who are not open to the concepts of charity or global responsibility. The intention to make the world a better place was what mattered, along with the acts of charity he could personally perform. When he returned to this life, he felt a little sad, possibly because he was no longer in the idyllic future. Or he may have been grieving about the coming calamity, sensing its inevitability at some level, as most of us do.

When he was awake, he described the vivid and powerful scenes, and the feelings and sensations he had experienced. This is one reason that I think this is not all imagination. Yet his excitement did not come close to matching mine, for I finally saw the implications. I had come to learn that past, present, and future are one and that what happens in the future can influence the present, just as the past influences it. That night I wrote: "We can go into the future if it's done wisely. The future, whether near or far, can be our guide. The future may be feeding back into the present to influence us now into making better choices and decisions. We can change what we're doing now based on feedback from the future. And that changes our futures in a more positive direction."

Think of what that means! As we have had limitless past lives, so will we have limitless future ones. Using our knowledge of what went before *and what is to come*, we may be able to shape the world's future and *our* futures. This ties into the ancient concept of karma: What you do, so shall you reap. If you plant better seeds, grow better crops, and perform better actions, your harvesting in the future will reward you.

Since then I have progressed many others. Some have progressed into their own lives, some into a global future. Science fiction, wish fulfillment, imagination—all these might explain what they saw, but so might the possibility that they were actually there. Perhaps the ultimate lesson I can draw from this lifetime is what the future holds and how we can all influence it. That knowledge, at least as much of it as I have now, will color my next lives and yours on our voyage toward immortality.

The future is born from the past. Nearly all my patients experience past life regressions before they journey into their future. This route paves the way for increased understanding and allows them to make wise choices in the present.

That the future is flexible and that we will be *present* in that future are the concepts that are addressed in this book. Compassion, empathy, nonviolence, patience, and spirituality are life lessons we must all learn. This book will show you why they are crucial through the examples of some of my most remarkable patients, and I will add some simple exercises to begin to teach you how to achieve them in this life. A few of you might actually experience regressions, but don't be disappointed if they don't occur. If you master the lessons, this life and your next lives will be happier, easier, emotionally richer, and more fulfilled. What is more, if all of us learn them, the future itself will be better for us cumulatively, since knowingly or not we are all striving to achieve the ultimate goal which is love.

CHAPTER 1

Immortality

E ACH OF US IS IMMORTAL.
     I don't mean simply that we pass on our genes, our beliefs, our mannerisms, and our "ways" to our children and they, in turn, to their children, though of course we do. Nor do I mean that our accomplishments—the work of art, the new way of making shoes, the revolutionary idea, the recipe for blueberry pie—live after us, though of course they do. I mean that the most important part of us, our soul, lives forever.

Sigmund Freud described the mind as functioning on different levels. Among them is what he called the unconscious mind, of which we are not aware, by definition, but which stores all our experience and directs us to act as we do, think as we do, respond as we do, feel as we do. Only by accessing the unconscious, he saw, can we learn who we are and, with that knowledge, be able to heal. Some people have written that that is what the soul is—Freud's unconscious. And in my work of regressing people—and, lately, progressing people—to their past and future lives so that they can more easily heal themselves, this is what I see, too: the working of the immortal soul.

I believe that each of us possesses a soul that exists after the death of the physical body and that it returns time and time again to other bodies in a progressive effort to reach a higher plane. (One of the questions that comes up frequently is "Where do the souls come from since there are so many more people now than when the world started?" I have posed this question to many patients, and the answer is always the same: This is not the only place where there are souls. There are many dimensions, many different levels of consciousness where there are souls. Why should we feel that we're the only place? There is no limit to energy. This is one school of many schools. Also, a few patients have told me that souls can split and have simultaneous experiences.) There is no empirical evidence for this; the soul does not have DNA, at least not the physical kind described by the Nobel Prize–winning scientists James Watson and Francis Crick. But the anecdotal evidence is overwhelming and to me unassailably conclusive. I have seen it virtually every day since Catherine took me with her to past times as disparate as Arabia in 1863 B.C. and Spain in A.D. 1756.

For example, there are Elizabeth and Pedro (in *Only Love Is Real*), lovers in former lives who came together again in this one; Linda (in *Through Time into Healing*), guillotined in Scotland, married in Italy centuries later to her present-day grandfather, and later still growing old in Holland, surrounded by her large and loving family; Dan, Laura, and Hope (in *Messages from the Masters*); and some four thousand others—some I've written about, most not—whose souls have journeyed through past lives, carrying the immortal part of them to the present. (Some of these patients could speak foreign languages in their past lives that they'd never learned or studied in this one, a phenomenon called xenoglossy and a remarkable "proof" that what they were reporting was true.)

When my patients remembered themselves in their other lives, the traumas that had brought them to see me in the first place were eased and in some cases cured. That is one of the soul's primary purposes: to progress toward healing.

If it were only I who had seen such cases, then you might be right in thinking I was hallucinating or had lost my mind, but Buddhists and Hindus have been accumulating past life cases for thousands of years. Reincarnation was written of in the New Testament until the time of Constantine, when the Romans censored it. Jesus himself may have believed in it, for he asked the Apostles if they recognized John the Baptist as Elijah returned; Elijah had lived nine hundred years before John. It is a fundamental tenet of Jewish mysticism; in some sects it was standard teaching until the early nineteenth century.

Hundreds of other therapists have taped thousands of past life sessions, and many of their patients' experiences have been verified. I myself have checked specific details and events recorded in Catherine's and others' past life memories—accurate details and events impossible to ascribe to false memory or fantasy. I no longer doubt that reincarnation is real. Our souls have lived before and will live again. That is our immortality.

Just before we die, our soul, that part of us which is aware when it leaves the body, pauses for a moment, floating. In that state it can differentiate color, hear voices, identify objects, and review the life it has just departed. This phenomenon is called an out-of-body experience, and it has been documented thousands of times, most famously by Elisabeth Kübler-Ross and Raymond Moody. Each of us experiences it when we die, but only a few have come back to present life to report on it.

One was reported to me (I mentioned it briefly in *Only Love Is Real*), not by the patient herself but by her cardiologist at Mount Sinai Medical Center in Miami, a scientist who is very academic and very grounded. The patient, an elderly diabetic, was hospitalized for medical tests. During her hospitalization she had a cardiac arrest (her heart stopped beating), and she became comatose. Doctors held out little hope. Nevertheless, they worked feverishly on her and called on her cardiologist for help.

He rushed into the intensive care unit and in so doing dropped his distinctive gold pen, which rolled across the room and under a window. During a short break in the resuscitation process, he retrieved it.

While the team worked on her, the woman reported later, she floated out of her body and watched the entire procedure from a point above the medicine cart, near that window. She watched with great concentration since it was she the doctors were working on. She longed to call out to them, to assure them that she was all right and that they didn't have to work so frantically, but she knew they couldn't hear her. When she tried to tap her cardiologist on the shoulder to tell him she was fine, her hand went right through him, and he felt nothing. She could see everything that was going on around her body and hear every word her doctors said, yet, to her frustration, nobody would listen to her.

The doctors' efforts succeeded. The woman returned to life.

"I watched the whole process," she told her cardiologist.

He was flabbergasted. "You couldn't have. You were unconscious. You were comatose!"

"That was a pretty pen you dropped," she said. "It must be very valuable."

"You saw it?"

"I just told you I did," she said and proceeded to describe the pen, the clothes the doctors and nurses wore, the succession of people who came in and out of the ICU, and what each did— things nobody could have known without having been there.

The cardiologist was still shaken days later when he told me about it. He confirmed that everything the woman related had indeed taken place and that her descriptions were accurate. Yet there was no question that she was unconscious; moreover, she had been blind for more than five years! Her *soul* had sight, not her body.

Since then the cardiologist has told me of dying patients who have seen familiar long-deceased people waiting to take them to the other side. These were patients who were not on medications of any kind and were therefore lucid. One described his grand-mother waiting patiently in a chair in his hospital room for his time to come. Another was visited by her child who had died in infancy. The cardiologist noted that among this population of his patients there was a calmness, a serenity about dying. He learned to tell his patients: "I'm very interested in what you feel and what you experience. No matter how strange or unusual it may seem, you're safe in talking about it to me." When they did, their fear of death decreased.

More commonly, those who are resuscitated report seeing light, often golden and at a distance, as though at the end of a tunnel. Andrea, a news reporter for a major television network, allowed me to regress her as a demonstration and described her life as a Great Plains farm woman in the nineteenth century. At the end of her long lifetime she floated above her body, watching it from afar. Then she felt she was being drawn up into a light, in her case a blue one, becoming increasingly distanced from her body and going toward a new life, one that was as yet unclear. This is a common, almost classic near death experience except that Andrea was describing the experience of someone in a past life—herself—who had been dead for more than one hundred years.

Where does the soul go after it leaves the body? I'm not sure; there may be no word for it. I call it another dimension, a higher level of consciousness or higher state of consciousness. The soul certainly exists outside of the physical body, and it makes connections not only to the other lifetimes of the person it just departed but to all other souls. We die physically, but this part of us is indestructible and immortal. The soul is timeless. Ultimately, there is probably just one soul, one energy. Many people call this God, while others call it love; again, the name doesn't matter.

I see the soul as a body of energy that blends with universal energy, then splits off again, intact, when it returns to a new life.

Before it merges with the One, it looks down on the body it has left and conducts what I call a life review, a review of the life just departed. The review is undertaken in a spirit of loving kindness and caring. It is not for punishment, it is for learning.

Your soul registers its experience. It feels the appreciation and gratitude of everyone you have helped and everyone you have loved in a heightened way now that it has left the body. Similarly, it feels the pain, anger, and despair of everyone you have hurt or betrayed, again magnified. In this way the soul learns not to do harmful things but to be compassionate.

Once the soul has finished its review, it seems to go further from your body, often finding the beautiful light as Andrea's ancestor did, though this may not happen immediately. It doesn't matter; the light is always there. Sometimes there are other souls around—you could call them masters or guides—who are very wise and help your soul on its journey toward the One. At some level your soul merges with the light, but it still retains its awareness so that it can continue to learn on the other side. It is a simultaneous merging with a greater light (at the end of the immortal journey, the merging will be complete), accompanied by feelings of indescribable bliss and joy, and the awareness that it remains individuated and still has lessons to learn, both on Earth and on the other side. Eventually—the time varies—the soul decides to come back in another body, and when it reincarnates, the sense of merging is lost. Some people believe there is a profound sadness at the separation from this glory, this bliss in the merging of energy and light, and it may be so.

On Earth, in the present, we are individuals, but individuation is an illusion characteristic of this plane, this dimension, this planet. Yes, we are here, as real and substantial as the chair on which you may be sitting as you read. But scientists know that a chair is just atoms, molecules, energy; it is a chair *and* it is energy. We are human, finite, *and* we are immortal.

I think that at the highest level all souls are connected. It is our illusion or grand delusion that we are individuated, separate.

Even as that pertains here, we are nevertheless connected to every other soul; thus, in a different sphere, we are all one. On this world our bodies are dense and physically heavy; they suffer from illness and disease. But in higher realms, I believe, no physical illness exists. In still higher realms there is nothing physical, only pure consciousness. And beyond that—and beyond that—in realms we cannot comprehend and where all souls are one, even time doesn't exist. This means that past, present, and future lives may be occurring simultaneously.

I'm a medical doctor and a psychiatrist, and healing is my life's passion. I believe we are each instinctively motivated toward spiritual healing and spiritual growth, toward understanding and compassion, toward evolution. I believe we move spiritually forward, not backward. The unconscious (or subconscious or superconscious mind or soul) has built within it a mechanism that steers it along a positive path of spiritual evolution. In other words, the soul *always, at all times, evolves toward health*. At a higher level, time is measured in lessons learned, though on Earth it is chronological. We live both in time and out of it. Our past and future lives converge in the present, and if they can induce us toward healing now so that our current lives are healthier and more spiritually fulfilled, we will make progress. The feedback loop is continuous, trying to get us to improve our future lives even as we live out this one.

I think many of us spend too much time worrying about what the higher levels of comprehension might be. The question is fascinating to contemplate, but our goal here is to heal ourselves as we are in our physical world. I see a lot of people, particularly New Age people, who aren't well grounded in this world—being right here, now. Progression in the areas of contemplation and meditation is important, but those who spend their lives in seclusion should understand that we are a social species and those who do not experience the joys of the physical, the pleasures of the senses, aren't learning the full lesson this present life has to teach them.

As I said, until recently I have only regressed patients so that they see and understand their past lives. Now I have begun to progress them into the future. But even if we study only our past lives, we can see how we have evolved within them. Each of our lives is a learning experience, and if we gain wisdom from our past lives, then through free will—conscious free will, that is, and the free will of the soul—we can affect the present.

Our souls choose our parents, for our impulse is to continue the learning process so we can proceed toward healing. We choose what we do in our present life for the same reason. We do not choose abusive parents, for no one wants to be abused. Yet some parents become abusive (it is their free will) and in a later life, or perhaps in this one, they will learn the lesson of compassion and stop that behavior.

I chose to come back as the son of Alvin and Dorothy Weiss, and to be a psychiatrist. In my previous life I was an underground Czech resistance fighter, killed in 1942 or '43. Perhaps the way I died led me to my present study of immortality; perhaps my desire to study and teach was a carryover from an earlier life as a priest in ancient Babylonia. Whatever, I chose to come back as Brian Weiss so I could maximize my personal learning and share it with others by becoming a healer. I selected my parents because they made it easy for me to learn. My father revered academics and wanted me to become a doctor. He was also interested in religion and taught me about Judaism, but he didn't force it. So I became a secular rabbi, a psychiatrist. My mother was loving and nonjudgmental. She gave me a sense of safety that in later life allowed me to risk my career and financial security by publishing *Many Lives, Many Masters*. Neither parent was spiritual in the New Age sense, nor did they believe in reincarnation. I chose them, it seems, because they offered me support and the freedom to go on the life path I eventually selected. Was anyone involved with me in that decision? I wonder. Spirits, guides, angels, all of them part of the one soul? I don't know.

True, some soul chose to come back as Saddam Hussein, another as Osama bin Laden. I believe they came back to maximize their learning opportunities, the same as you and me. They did not choose to come back initially to do harm, to cause violence and blow up other people and become terrorists. They came back to *resist* that urge, probably because they had succumbed to it in previous lifetimes. They came back for a kind of field test in this school we live in, and they failed miserably.

This is all speculation, of course, but I believe their souls came back to inhabit them in an effort to find alternatives to violence, prejudice, and hatred. (The abusive parent's soul comes back for the same reason.) They amassed money and power, and faced the choice of violence or compassion, prejudice or teaching, hatred or love. This time we know their decision. They will have to come back again, face the consequences of their actions, face the choices again, until they are able to move forward.

Students ask me why anyone would choose to come back to live in a rat-infested slum in Bogotá or Harlem. The Buddhist monks I've met, the entourage of the Dalai Lama, laugh at the question because they see life as a stage performance. The man in the slum is just a role; in the next lifetime the same actor will appear as a prince. I believe we choose to come into a rat-infested apartment because we have to understand what it is like to be poor; in other lifetimes we will be rich. We must be rich, poor, male, female, healthy, sickly, big, small, strong, and weak. If in one lifetime I'm wealthy and someone else is living as I once did, in the slums of Bogotá, then I will want to help that person because it will be a step in my own growth.

There are two vital elements at work here. First, we cannot learn everything in one lifetime. That doesn't matter because there are numerous lifetimes to come. Second, each time we come back, it is to be healed.

* * *

Our lives are a series of steps up the evolutionary scale. Where are we, then, when we are completely healed, when we reach the top of the staircase? Probably at the highest spiritual level, which some call heaven, others nirvana.

I believe that our planet was created as a place to experience emotions, sensations, feelings, and relationships. Here we can be in love and feel great pleasure and joy. We can smell flowers, touch a baby's skin, see the glory of a landscape, hear the music of the wind. *That* was the intent. What a classroom!

In the next years our great test will be whether we want to honor this school or destroy it, as modern technology has made it possible for us to do. I'm not sure our free will can make that choice; it may be our destiny. If a higher mind, the Oneness, decides that our planet is worth preserving, then it won't be destroyed. If it does not, and we vaporize the world, our souls will nevertheless endure; they would find another school.

But it may not be as beautiful as our world; it may not be as physical.

Our souls are all the same age, which is ageless, but some souls advance more quickly than others. Saddam Hussein may be a third grader, while the Dalai Lama is in graduate school. In the end we will all graduate to the One. How quickly we progress depends on our free will.

The free will I am writing about here isn't the same as our soul's ability to choose our parents and our circumstances. Rather, it is human will, and we are in control of it on Earth. I distinguish it from destiny, which often brings us together with another for good or for ill.

It is free will that lets us choose what we eat, our cars, our clothes, our vacations. Free will allows us to select our partners as

well, though it is probably destiny that draws us to them and they
to us. I met Carole, my wife, in the Catskill Mountains; I was a
busboy, and she was a guest at the hotel where I was working.
Destiny. The course of our relationship—like the course of hundreds of millions of other relationships—depended on our free
will. We chose to date, and we chose to marry.

Similarly, we can choose to increase our capacity to love or be
compassionate; we can choose to perform the little acts of kindness that bring us internal satisfaction; we can choose generosity
over selfishness, respect over prejudice. In every aspect of our lives
we can choose to make the loving decision, and by doing so, our
souls will evolve.

John E. Mack, M.D., the Pulitzer Prize–winning author and
professor of psychiatry at Harvard Medical School, points out that

> we are now witnessing a coming together of science,
> psychology, and spirituality after centuries of ideological
> and disciplinary fragmentation. Both modern physics
> and depth psychology are revealing to us a universe in
> which . . . all that we can perceive around us is connected
> by resonances, both physical and nonphysical, that can
> make the possibility of universal justice, truth and love
> more than just a utopian fantasy.
>
> At the heart of this possibility lie what in the
> Western secular world are called "non-ordinary" states
> of consciousness, but in the world's great religious
> traditions is variously called primary religious feeling,
> mystical oneness, connection with the ground of being,
> or universal love. . . . At the heart of these states of
> consciousness or being is a potential extension of the
> self beyond its usual boundaries.

I would substitute "soul" for "self" and add that the boundaries exceed the measurable universe.

* * *

It has taken me twenty-four years to reach the simple truth at the core of this book. We are immortal. We are eternal. Our souls will never die. This being so, we should start acting as if we know that immortality is our blessing. Or, to put it more simply, *we should prepare for immortality*—here, now, today and tomorrow and each day for the rest of our lives. If we prepare, our souls will move up the evolutionary scale, come closer to healing, come closer to the higher state. If we don't, we will recycle our present lives—in effect, march in place—and postpone to a future life the mastering of the lesson we might have learned in this one.

How do we prepare? How do immortal people act? In this life we prepare by learning how to have better relationships; how to be more loving, more compassionate; how to be healthier physically, emotionally, and spiritually; how to help others; how to enjoy this world and yet advance its evolution, advance its healing. By preparing for immortality we will quiet present fears, feel better about ourselves, and grow spiritually. And we will be healing our future lives at the exact same moment.

Now, thanks to the progressions that my patients have experienced and reported back to me, we can see the results of our present behavior and thus shape it for the future. If we can accelerate the healing process, the evolutionary process, that is the most therapeutic action we can take, the best thing we can do, not only for our own souls but for everyone in the world. This is what I have learned from my patients.

CHAPTER 2

George:
Anger Management

ANGER MANAGEMENT is one of the skills we can learn now in order to avoid repetitions of violence in our lives to come. The following case history is of a man I treated before I began progressing some of my patients. Had he been able to see what lay in the years ahead, his treatment might have gone more quickly.

George Skulnick was doing his best to destroy himself. Despite a history of a heart attack and high blood pressure, he was over-weight, smoked heavily, worked too hard, canceled vacations at the last moment, and misused his heart medications by either forgetting to take them or, to compensate, by taking too many at a time. He had already suffered one serious heart attack and was primed for another.

His cardiologist, Barbara Tracy, recommended that he see me for stress management.

"George is a tough case," Barbara had warned. "Beware of explosions."

And now here he was in my office with his wife, a woman in

her mid-forties who looked at me with what I took to be pleading eyes.

"Betty will sit in the waiting room," George said, "in case you need her."

"If you wouldn't mind," I said gently, turning to her.

"Not at all." She gave me one last pleading look and then left the office, closing the door behind her.

George was a squat, solid, powerful-looking man with massive arms, too great a stomach, and surprisingly spindly legs, a nonathletic Babe Ruth. His moon face was florid; capillaries had burst around his nose, hinting at heavy drinking. I judged him to be nearly sixty, though it turned out he was only fifty-two.

"You're the reincarnation doctor," he said—a fact, not a question.

"I am."

"I don't believe in that crap."

If he was trying to unnerve me, it didn't work. "Many people don't."

"Dr. Tracy said you practiced something called regression therapy."

"Yes. Often it leads the patient back to past lives."

"Bullsh—" He stopped himself and raised a hand. "Don't get me wrong. I'm game for anything if it'll prevent another attack."

Actually, George had once reported a near death experience to Barbara. During his heart attack he had felt himself rising out of his body toward a cloud of blue light. While he was floating, he became aware of a thought: Everything was going to be all right. This knowledge calmed him, and he wanted to tell his family about it. From his vantage point he could see where his wife and two children were. They were extremely anxious, and he wanted to reassure them but couldn't. He glanced away for another view of his body, and when he looked back, he could see they weren't paying any attention to him. It was as if it was years after his death. This event persuaded him to come to me.

"Why don't we decide what to do after I find out more about you," I said. "Dr. Tracy says you're in the construction business."

"Skulnick Contractors. We specialize in factories, warehouses, and office buildings. You must have seen our signs. They're all over Miami."

I had indeed.

"It's a lot of headaches," he continued. "Constant pres-sure. If I don't oversee every site personally, someone's sure to screw up."

"What happens if they do?"

His eyes flashed. "I get angry."

I knew from Barbara that rage was the greatest danger George faced, a knife poised at his heart. "Tell me about the anger," I said.

"I lose control. I'm a screamer. My face gets red, and I feel my heart pumping and about to explode." His breath quickened even as he talked. "I want to lash out, hit somebody, *kill* somebody. I get so mad."

"What about when you're with your wife, your family?"

"It's just as bad, maybe worse. Sometimes I'll be furious at somebody in the office, have a few drinks on my way home, and come in looking for a fight. Dinner not ready? *Pow!* Haven't done your homework? *Whap!*" He lowered his head to his palms. "They're terrified of me. I don't really hit them, of course. But there may come a time—"

"I see. Maybe we can find out where the rage comes from."

He raised his head. "My father, I suppose. He was a screamer, and he drank, too."

"That might explain it," I said, "but maybe there's more."

"Something that happened in a past life?"

I shrugged. "It's possible."

"And you think regression will help?"

"I believe it's important for you, yes, though I could help you through traditional psychotherapy, and you might prefer that.

The fact that you had a near death episode makes me think you'll regress easily. And if it's unpleasant for you or painful or too intense, I'll know immediately and we'll stop."

He was silent for a moment. Then: "You use hypnosis, right?"

"Yes."

"If I'm hypnotized, how will you know if I want to stop?"

"You'll tell me."

"From my other life?"

"Exactly."

I could see a *yeah, sure* form in his brain, but all he said was "Come on. Let's give it a try."

In *Through Time into Healing* I wrote the following:

> Hypnosis is the main technique I use to help patients access past life memories. . . . One goal of hypnosis, as well as meditation, is to access the subconscious. . . . In the subconscious mind mental processes occur without our conscious perception of them. We experience moments of intuition, wisdom, and creativity when these processes flash into our conscious awareness.
>
> The subconscious is not limited by our imposed boundaries of logic, space, and time. It can remember everything, from any time. . . . It can transcend the ordinary to touch upon a wisdom far beyond our everyday capabilities. Hypnosis accesses the wisdom of the subconscious in a focused way in order to achieve healing. We are in hypnosis whenever the usual relationship between the conscious and subconscious mind is reconfigured so that the subconscious plays a more dominant role. . . .
>
> When you are hypnotized, you are *not* asleep. Your conscious mind is always aware of what you are experiencing while you are hypnotized. Despite the deep sub-

conscious contact, your mind can comment, criticize, and censor. You are always in control of what you say. Hypnosis is *not* a "truth serum." You do not enter a time machine and suddenly find yourself transported to another time and place with no awareness of the present. . . .

It may sound as though it requires a great deal of skill to reach these deeper levels of hypnosis. However, each of us experiences them with ease every day as we pass through the state between wakefulness and sleeping known as the hypnagogic state. . . .

Listening to someone's guiding voice aids in focusing concentration and helps a patient to reach a deeper level of hypnosis and relaxation. There is no danger in hypnosis. No person I have ever hypnotized has become "stuck" in the hypnotic state. You can emerge from a state of hypnosis whenever you want. No one has ever violated his or her moral and ethical principles. No one has involuntarily acted like a chicken or a duck. No one can control you. You are in control.

In hypnosis, your mind is always aware and observing. This is why people who may be deeply hypnotized and actively involved in a childhood or past life sequence of memories are able to answer the therapist's questions, speak their current life language, know the geographical places they are seeing, and even know the year, which usually flashes before their inner eyes or just appears in their minds. The hypnotized mind, always retaining an awareness and a knowledge of the present, puts the childhood or past life memories into context. If the year 1900 flashes, and you find yourself building a pyramid in ancient Egypt, you *know* that the year is B.C., even if you don't see those actual letters.

This is also why a hypnotized patient, finding himself a peasant fighting in a medieval European war, for example, can recognize people from that past lifetime whom he knows in his current life. This is why he can speak modern English, compare the crude weapons of that time with those he might have seen or used in this lifetime, give dates, and so on.

His present-day mind is aware, watching, commenting. He can always compare the details and events with those of his current life. He is the movie's observer and its critic and usually its star at the same time. And all the while, he can remain in the relaxed, hypnotic state.

Hypnosis puts the patient in a state that holds great potential for healing by giving the patient access to the subconscious mind. To speak metaphorically, it puts the patient in the magical forest that holds the healing tree. But if hypnosis lets the patient into that healing country, it is the regression process that is the tree that holds the sacred berries he or she must eat to heal.

Regression therapy is the mental act of going back to an earlier time, whenever that time may be, in order to retrieve memories that may still be negatively influencing a patient's present life and that are probably the source of the patient's symptoms. Hypnosis allows the mind to short-circuit conscious barriers to tap this information, including those barriers that prevent patients from consciously accessing their past lives.

I would escort George into that forest, maintaining my role as therapist by making no effort to suggest or influence what berries he might find on the tree, by keeping my voice calm and soothing to ensure his comfort and relaxation, by asking only those questions that would allow him to further describe what he was seeing, by showing no surprise, by making no moral judgments, by giving no interpretation but instructing him in selected instances—in short, by acting as a guide.

He sat on a small, comfortable couch. I faced him from my chair. "Relax," I said. "Close your eyes. . . ." And we began.

Neither of us knew what he would find.

"I'm an innkeeper," he said, "a German innkeeper. I'm lying on a bed in a room upstairs, our bedroom. It's the Middle Ages. I'm an old man, over seventy, and very weak, though recently I was strong. I can see myself clearly. I'm unkempt, my clothes are soiled. I'm sick. My once powerful arms are thin now. My back muscles, with which I could lift boulders, have atrophied. I have barely enough strength to sit up." He looked at me from a distance of seven centuries and bowed his head. "I have no heart."

His family surrounded him. "I was unkind to them all. Mean to my wife. Mean to my children. I neglected them, drank, and had affairs with other women. But they were dependent on me, couldn't leave me, even though I abused them. My rages were violent. They were afraid of me."

Recently, he had suffered a stroke or heart attack, and now it was he who was dependent on them. But despite his abusiveness and neglect, they took care of him with compassion, even with love. His wife in his present life was his son in his past life, and his daughter in his present life was his wife in his past one.

(Such permutations are common. Those who are important in a present life were important in past ones and remain with us.)

His family tended to him tirelessly and without complaint, for he was too sick to do anything for himself. Eventually, his body, ruined by years of excessive drinking, gave out, and he floated above his grieving family, looking down on them, feeling guilty that he had treated them so abysmally.

It is at the time of the death of the body that one conducts a life review, and he reported that guilt was what he felt most, guilt for a life misspent.

"Let go of your guilt," I told him. "There's no need for it anymore. The family is fine, and guilt is holding you back."

Together we reviewed his life as an innkeeper. What lessons could he draw from it? He was still hypnotized, still in the inn, still aware of the instant he died. His thoughts were expressed in choppy sentences, but the feelings behind them were clear and pure.

"There's great foolishness in danger and violence," he said. "Bodies are fragile and temporary. There is safety in love and compassion. All families need nurturing and sustenance. I needed to nurture them, just as they nurtured me. The greatest power is the power of love."

All this he reported with the force of revelation. When he finished, he seemed exhausted, so I brought him gently back to the present, and we were able to discuss his insights, what he had found when he went back. He left feeling dazed—the first regression is unfailingly powerful—and promised to return the following week.

When he left, I jotted a note to myself: "Can see future life seeds planted here, to his current life. Again a heart attack. Again abuse of his family. A similar pattern. There's a lesson coming up."

I looked forward to George's return.

He was a seventeen-year-old soldier the next time I regressed him, fighting for his country, France, during World War I. His left arm was blown off in an explosion, and when he experienced this, he clutched his arm and reported feeling pain. But the pain disappeared, for he realized that he had died from his wounds. Again, in the instant of that death, he floated above his body and was able to see himself at another time in the same life. He was no longer a soldier but an observer, detached from the events he was describing. Now he was a boy, no more than ten, living a hardworking but peaceful life on a farm, with two loving parents and a younger sister who idolized him. There were horses, cows, and chickens on the farm. It was not an eventful prior life, this life before the war.

I wondered if the pain in his left arm correlated with the heart attack he had experienced both earlier and very recently, but I couldn't be sure. Sometimes it is simple to see a connection between past and present lives, but in this case I didn't get a good follow-up.

I didn't have a chance to think about it for long because suddenly he became extremely agitated. He had connected his French life to another. (It is unusual when this happens; normally, a regression leads to one lifetime, though the patient will often cover different times and events in that same life.) Now he was a warrior, a Mongol or Tatar, living in Russia or Mongolia—he couldn't be sure. It was some nine hundred years ago. Fearsomely strong, a master horseman, he roamed the steppes, killing his enemies and amassing great wealth. The people he killed were often innocent young men, many of them farmers who had been conscripted into the army against their will, like the French boy he would eventually become. He killed hundreds during his lifetime and died an old man, without any of the regret he experienced two hundred years later when he was the German innkeeper. He himself did not suffer. He learned no lessons; those would come in later lives. The life review he did as the innkeeper seemed to be the first time he experienced contrition.

His Mongol experience showed me something I had recently begun to figure out: Learning about the consequences of your actions is not necessarily an immediate thing. He would have to go through other violent lifetimes before he could feel what he had caused. How many lifetimes I couldn't be sure; I could only count the number he reported.

Perhaps he had been killed in World War I as retribution for his violent life as a warrior. Perhaps his innkeeper contrition was not enough. Perhaps if he had changed prior to his acts of violence, he would not have come back to be killed in France. Perhaps he would have lived a long life on the farm. We discussed all this when I brought him out of hypnosis. I think he was telling me that if he had not been so violent in his past lives, he wouldn't be so violent in his present life. He had gone from remorseless killer to abusive innkeeper to French soldier, killed before he had a chance for a full life, to a successful businessman who was still raging and had severe heart problems and high blood pressure.

That day I wrote two notes: "The value of empathy. He had to feel what he had caused" and "The heart is connecting these lifetimes." What would come next?

This time he was a thin, gay Japanese man in his thirties, living in the late nineteenth century. He told me he had an affair of the heart; he had fallen in love with a much younger man. There was no way to get the young man's love, he felt, other than seducing him, so that is what he set out to do. Alcohol was the means. He took his beloved to a room and plied him with liquor. Half against the young man's will, they became lovers that night.

The young man was ashamed, embarrassed, and humiliated. Homosexuality was a dishonorable, forbidden act in his culture; the young man was particularly mortified that he had allowed himself to be taken. His reaction was rage. He arrived at their next rendezvous with a knife or sword and plunged it into the older man's chest. George was too thin and weak to resist. My patient died instantly.

In his life review, the themes of hatred, anger, impulsive rage, and alcohol were all present. He should have been more patient, George realized. He did not have to seduce the younger man but could have waited for a willing partner. He was not judging his homosexuality; his sin was in interfering with someone else's free will by manipulating him.

A more subtle connection centered on weight. For all his strength, George was obese, which added to his risk of heart attack. Sometimes people put on and maintain weight as a protection. This is common with women who have been abused or raped; symbolically, they are trying to prevent that violence from recurring. And here was George, a rapist who was also a victim of

violence. His obesity seemed to stem from that life and from another, not this one. Once George understood this, dieting became
easier.

I wrote: "His past life scar—maybe from the knife wound—
cardiac susceptibility in the future?" I couldn't be sure, but frequently we come back with wounds or weaknesses in the areas of
the body that were the site of mortal wounds or damage in a past
life. In George's case the connection seemed likely.

By this time George was able to go very deep. He seemed
shaken by his experiences and inspired by them.

In 1981 when my patient Catherine was in a deep hypnotic
state and remembering the significant lessons from her past lives,
she brought back messages from "the Masters." Now I asked
George when he stayed in a deeper state, "Is there anything more?
Are there any other messages for you, any other information or
wisdom for you to take back?"

I took down all he said as though I were taking dictation:
"The earth life is a gift. It is a school to learn how love manifests
in the physical dimensions where bodies and emotions exist. But
the school has many playgrounds, and those need to be used. The
physical life is meant to be enjoyed. This is one reason you have
been given the senses. Be good people. Have fun and enjoy yourselves. Enjoy the simple yet abundant pleasures of life while not
harming other people or other things, like nature."

When he left I wrote: "When George awoke, he knew these
messages were very important to him because he didn't have any
fun in his present life, and these are simple things about why
we're here. There are playgrounds here, too. It's not all work and
serious. 'Be good people' meant to be compassionate and caring
at all levels."

When he came to his next session, George told me about a
miraculous dream. Whatever doubts he had about regression
therapy had disappeared. He was excited, vibrant. The messages
he had learned took the form of a person, a spiritual being
bathed in the blue light he had seen during his first regression.

The person in the blue light told him he needed to love himself more and that Earth people needed to take care of one another, not harm others. He received instructions, he told me, though he wasn't able to go into much detail. They were instructions meant for him, he knew, but concerned humanity at all levels. He needed to communicate better, to explain his thoughts and actions, rather than just lashing out. Be more gentle, the spirit said. Don't do harm to others.

George told me that there was a hierarchy of spirits and that the one who visited him in his dream wasn't necessarily at the highest level. There are other places and other dimensions that are even higher and do not belong to the Earth. Still, we have to learn the lessons of the Masters because the important thing was to progress, he said. While this was not as cogent or encompassing as the messages that Catherine had delivered, I was moved by it. Once again it was a case of patient leading doctor.

Different connections were evident in George's next regression. This time his life was as a southern slave woman in the early eighteenth century. George was married to a particularly brutal man. The husband in the black woman's life was also George's father in his present life. In the early life George's husband beat his wife so savagely that he broke her legs, rendering her paralyzed.

In this life George's father was a source of great strength and support, particularly in George's childhood, which was marked by arthritis in George's knees. But George's father was a frightening authoritarian figure, given to the same kind of rages that George would later repeat, and the boy quickly learned that to accomplish things away from his father's influence, he would have to "stand up for himself," an obvious correlation to his life as a slave.

Independence and strength became the hallmarks of George's pre-heart-attack life, and he carried them with him, perhaps too single-mindedly, even after he got out of the hospital.

The lesson George needed to learn in this lifetime was balance; he had to combine authority with the ability to listen to others, to take suggestions as well as give orders.

He regressed briefly into another life, of which he just saw glimpses. He was a Stone Age man clothed in animal skins, with hairy hands and feet. But he died very young—of starvation. Here was another explanation for his excessive weight in this life: People close to starvation, such as those who died in the Holocaust, often become overweight when reincarnated, needing the weight as reassurance they would never be hungry again.

I put his past lives in chronological order: Stone Age man, Mongol warrior, innkeeper in the Middle Ages, slave woman with paralyzed legs, murdered Japanese gay man, and Frenchman dying for his country. Surely there were many additional lives as well, but he did not get to them in our sessions and perhaps never would. His blue spirit told him that we see the past lifetimes that are important to this one.

"Learning keeps happening on the other side, too," George told me, now an "expert," and I was pleased at his positiveness. "You develop skills. You work on your talents. It doesn't stop."

There were consistent themes in all the lives he remembered—violence and anger, physical pain, abusiveness, constant threat of death—that were paralleled in his present life. When George put the past lives together, it became obvious to him that his present-day lifestyle was deadly. He was drinking too much. His blood pressure needed to be controlled. He could have another heart attack. His rages put him in danger of a stroke.

All this took nearly two years of intense therapy (with periodic sessions thereafter), but as he joined these insights with other therapeutic tools I gave him, such as relaxation CDs, I had the pleasure of watching him begin to shift. He was able to relax more without doing formal meditation (something I had recommended but that he would not do). He reported communicating better with the people in his office; he said he was better able to listen and to accept setbacks without "going ballistic." Even when he did get angry, the periods were briefer and less violent. He was able to relax from time to time; he would put on one of my CDs in his office during lunch hour and tell his secretary to make sure he wasn't interrupted. He started to play golf and go fishing again, and attend Florida Marlins baseball games.

Physically, George was getting better, too. His blood pressure went down, and his heart function improved. He began to exercise, he drank less, and he ate healthier foods, all in concert with his wife. Sometimes I would bring her into our sessions, where she verified his progress with a gratitude that was as heartfelt as his. It was the same with their children; he was becoming a father, a friend, and a guide, not a dictator.

One change led to another, and soon there was a progression of changes—what we call a synergistic loop. Success followed success.

"I had glimpses of the other side," he told me. "I saw myself in a future life as a beloved teacher to many children. It was a very happy life. I was very content. The skills I learned were ones I could bring back to my physical life here. And I saw another world, just glimpses of it. Crystalline structures and lights and people—you know, like light beams."

I was astonished. As I say, this was before I was purposely taking people into the future. His vision, I thought then, might have been a metaphor, a symbol for what his present-day soul wished for, or it might have been nothing more than a dream influenced by our work on his past. Still, perhaps what he saw was true.

At the end of our last session I wrote: "He has healed the spiritual heart as well as the physical heart." His cardiologist, Barbara Tracy, confirmed the physical part, and I knew that George was hopeful now. Life was suddenly important to him. Spirituality became part of his psychological makeup. Family mattered. Friends mattered. Coworkers mattered. Pleasure, too.

He was prepared for the next stage in his evolution. When George's body dies and his soul is ready to return, I am convinced his new life will be at a higher level; it will almost surely be gentler than the lives he has led. Had he not revisited and understood the lessons of his past lives, it would have taken him longer to reach the stage he is in now. He might have had to spend several more lives in an angry, violent state before he learned for himself the truths his regressions had shown him. His therapy terminated, and I no longer see him as a patient. Should he care to, I'd welcome the chance to progress him, not for therapeutic purposes but for us to see what his nonviolent next life—next lives—will be like.

George's present life was changed by his renunciation of anger and violence, his predominant issues. Other patients' present and past lives demonstrate how change is possible in a dozen different aspects of life and, by extrapolation, in hundreds more. It is rare that a person will master more than one lesson in one lifetime, though residual attention is often paid to others. For purposes of the book I have segregated the lessons into different discrete areas, though they often overlap and evolution in one can lead to evolution in others. The histories you are about to read are remarkable examples of people evolving toward new lives that take them to higher planes and will eventually lead to the highest plane of all.

CHAPTER 3

Victoria, Evelyn, and Michelle: Health

S A PHYSICIAN and psychiatrist my mission is to heal physical and emotional illness, sometimes separately but more often simultaneously since the mind affects the body's health, and the body the mind's. I am aware of the concept of "spiritual health," but to me the soul is always healthy. Indeed, the soul is perfect. When people talk about healing the soul, I don't know what they mean. It is our distance from being soulful that makes us feel the soul needs to be healed.

Poor health tends to make narcissists of us, and narcissism makes us blind to compassion, empathy, anger management, and patience—all the elements that, when mastered, will lead us higher up the evolutionary scale toward immortality. Often, if we are sick, we can think of nothing but the sickness, and there is little chance for progress. Thus in this chapter, I write about physical illness and diseases, and diseased states of mind—phobias, fears, depression, anxiety—and how to alleviate them. Do past lives have an impact on them? Absolutely. Do future lives also have an effect? More and more—the evidence continues to accumulate—I believe they do.

I am about to introduce you to two remarkable people, Victoria and Evelyn, the first with a cancer that made every day a time in hell, the other with such profound anxiety that an outwardly successful life was actually made virtually unmanageable. I cured Victoria by bringing her into her past lives; I've helped Evelyn by showing her the future.

By this time I'm used to amazing regressions, astonishing revelations, but Victoria's case filled me with a sense of the miraculous I had not often experienced since I first met Catherine twenty-four years ago.

Victoria is a physicist living in Manhattan, a renowned member of the Academy of Arts and Sciences. I met her when she came up to me at the start of a five-day workshop at the Omega Institute, a healing and learning center in Rhinebeck, New York. She told me that for the past sixteen years she had been experiencing severe back pain caused by a cancer that multiple operations and a series of chemotherapy and radiation treatments had been unable to cure. She handed me a file on her condition several inches thick. Her pain was unremitting; she described it as being like the relentless bombardment of an abscessed tooth. At night she had to take high doses of a morphine-like drug because the pain was so severe, but during the day she endured the agony so she could continue to work with a clear mind. Though not old— she was in her mid-fifties—her hair had turned gray from the pain. She didn't like the way it looked so she dyed it black.

Victoria had stopped taking her medicines a few days before the workshop, she averred, so she could concentrate on my lectures. But now she asked, "How can I last five days without medicine? I'll have to go home in an ambulance."

"Do your best," I said, "but I'll understand if you have to leave."

She stayed for all the sessions and at their end approached me with her report. It was so important that I asked her to share it with the group. During the week, she had experienced several regressions, all covering the same life, which took place near

Jerusalem at the time of Jesus. She was a poor male peasant, a powerful man with huge arms and shoulders, but spiritually sensitive and fond of birds and animals. He lived in a wooden house by the side of the road with his wife and daughter, bothering no one. Victoria recognized the daughter; she was her daughter now. One day, the peasant found a mourning dove that had broken its wing, and knelt to care for it. A Roman soldier, marching with an elite corps of the palace guard, was annoyed by this man blocking his path, and kicked him savagely in the back, breaking several vertebrae. Others of the corps set fire to his house, killing his wife and child. The peasant's bitterness and hatred of the Romans burned bright within him. From that moment on, he trusted no one. His back never healed.

In despair, broken physically and emotionally, he moved close to the main temple within the walls of Jerusalem where he lived in a lean-to, existing on the vegetables he was able to grow. He was unable to work, getting around only by leaning on a sturdy walking stick and his one animal, a donkey. People thought he was senile, but he was merely old and broken. News of a rabbi who was becoming famous as a healer caught his attention, and he traveled a great distance to hear a sermon by this man—it was the Sermon on the Mount—expecting not to be healed or comforted in any way, but curious all the same. The rabbi's followers were appalled at the sight of the peasant and shooed him away. He hid behind a bush and was able to meet Yeshi's eyes.* "It was like looking into bottomless pits filled with endless compassion," Victoria told me.

Yeshua said to the peasant, "Do not go far," and he obeyed for the rest of the day.

The encounter brought the peasant not healing but hope. He went back to his lean-to, inspired by the rabbi's sermon, which he found "ringing and true."

---

*Victoria called him Yeshi, the diminutive of Yeshua, the rabbi's Aramaic name. Jesus, the name we know him by, is Greek. Victoria had never heard the name Yeshi until she encountered it in her regression.

When the rabbi was about to return to Jerusalem, the peasant became stricken with anxiety. He knew Yeshua was in a dangerous situation, having heard rumors of what the hated Romans had planned for him. He tried to reach the rabbi to warn him, but he was too late. The next time they communicated, Yeshua was struggling under the weight of a huge wooden beam on his way to being crucified. He was, the peasant knew, extremely dehydrated. Amazed at his own courage, he reached out to Yeshua with a cloth soaked in water to wet his mouth, but Yeshua had already passed by. The peasant felt terrible, but then Yeshua looked back at him, again with infinite compassion in his eyes despite his physical struggle, dehydration, and fatigue. Though Yeshua did not speak, the peasant became aware of his words that etched themselves telepathically in his mind: "It's all right. This was meant to be." Yeshua walked on. The peasant followed him to Calvary, to the crucifixion.

Victoria's next memory was of herself as the peasant standing alone in the pouring rain, sobbing, minutes after Yeshua's death on the cross. Yeshua was the only one he trusted since his family was killed, and now the rabbi, too, was dead. Suddenly he felt what Victoria described as "electricity" at the top of his head. It shot down his spine, and he became aware that his back was straight; he was no longer hunchbacked or crippled. He was strong again.

"Look," Victoria cried in the present. "Look!"

She began to dance, swiveling her own hips, completely pain free. There had been no witnesses when the peasant stood straight; two thousand years later, everyone at the conference watched Victoria dance. Some were crying. My own eyes filled with tears. Sometimes when I go over my notes as I review a case, I forget the sense of magic, the sense of mystery and awe that regressions evoke in me, but now it was palpable. This was not hypnotic suggestion. That she had severe vertebral damage and cartilage loss was documented by the MRIs and other tests reported in the file she gave me.

I remember thinking, "How will this physicist, this woman of science, incorporate what has just happened into her life?" It was an intellectual question that might in time be answered. For the moment, as I watched her, all I could feel was her joy.

Something more wondrous was yet to happen.

In *Only Love Is Real,* I wrote briefly about a past life memory of my own. I was a young man from a very wealthy family living in Alexandria some two thousand years ago. I loved to travel and roamed the deserts of northern Egypt and southern Judea, often investigating the caves where the Essenes and other spiritual groups lived at the time. In fact, my family contributed to their well-being. During one journey I met a man somewhat younger than I who was exceptionally bright, and we camped and traveled together for about a month. He soaked up the teachings of these spiritual communities much faster than I did. Though we became good friends, eventually we went our separate ways, I to visit a synagogue near the Great Pyramids.

I did not relate the rest of this story at that time because it was extremely personal, and I did not want people to think I wrote out of self-congratulation: "Dr. Weiss in the time of Jesus." You'll see shortly why I do so now, for it is Victoria's story, not mine.

I saw my companion again in Jerusalem, where I often traveled because my family conducted much of their business there. I experienced myself in that storied city as a scholar, not a businessman, though I was still wealthy. By this time I had affected an immaculately trimmed salt-and-pepper beard and wore an extravagant robe, my own "coat of many colors." I saw it then, as I see it now, vividly.

At the time there was a traveling rabbi who was able to inspire huge groups of people and thus was a threat to Pontius Pilate, who placed him under a death sentence. I merged with the crowd gathered to see this person on his way to execution, and when I looked into his eyes, I knew that I had found my friend, but it was too late to even attempt to save him. All I could do was watch when he walked by, though I was later able to financially support some of his followers and his family.

I was thinking of this as Victoria, very much in the present and still exhilarated, was talking, so I only half-heard her when she said, "I saw you there."

"Where?" I asked.

"In Jerusalem. When Jesus was on his way to the cross. You were someone powerful."

A thrill went up my spine like fire along a fuse. "How did you know it was me?"

"By the expression in your eyes. It's the same expression I see in them now."

"What was I wearing?"

"A robe. It was sand colored with vivid burgundy piping, very elegant. You weren't one of the authorities, not one of Pilate's men, but I knew you had money because of the robe and because your salt-and-pepper beard was so neatly trimmed, unlike most of the people's. Oh, it was you, Brian! No doubt about it." Both of us felt goosebumps, and we looked at each other in wonder.

A psychiatrist might say, "Well, that's projection. You were teaching at Omega, an authority figure and a healer, and her pain is gone, so naturally she'd believe she saw you in her regression." True, but she described the robe, the beard, my appearance, the scene, and the situation exactly as I had seen it many years ago in my own regression. I had told only three people the full story of that regression; in no way could she have known what I looked like or what I was wearing.

There is something extremely remarkable going on here; to me it is inexplicable. It goes beyond health and healing into the realm of the transcendental. "This was meant to be," Jesus the healer told her. I sense these are important words, but I'm not sure how to interpret them.

She called me the night after the conference ended, still

shaken. Both of us, twin scientists, realized that her vision of Jesus had been validated. For some reason that neither of us understood, we had been taken beyond our science to two points where we had been destined to meet so that she might heal. It was neither accident nor fantasy that she saw me in Jerusalem; it meant that two thousand years later I was to be the instrument of her healing.

I asked her to keep in touch with me, and we speak regularly. She still moves without pain and can swivel her hips with the best of them. When she went back to her hairdresser, he marveled that her hair had kept its dye so well—and then realized that it had *grown in* black, its natural color. Her internist was, she said, "flabbergasted" by her ability to walk and dance without pain. And in October her pharmacist called her, concerned because she had not renewed her prescription for pain medication. "I don't need it anymore," she told him and, amazed at all that had happened, began to weep. "I'm fine."

Evelyn worked in mergers and acquisitions, meaning that she helped effectuate the merging of two companies or the sale of one to another. When the companies were large, there were often hundreds of millions of dollars involved, and the fees paid to the company that Evelyn worked for routinely came to seven figures. Evelyn was paid a substantial salary, which was often doubled or tripled by her year-end bonus, a reward for bringing in new business.

She was in her mid-thirties, slim, physically attractive, with black hair cropped short, almost a cliché of the young woman executive. Her clothes reflected her success: a Chanel suit and handbag, a Hermès scarf, shoes by Gucci, a Rolex watch, and a diamond necklace. Yet when I looked into her eyes—not easy since they darted away from me when she became conscious of my gaze—I could see sadness. The light was in the diamonds at her neck, not in her expression.

"I need help," she said the moment we shook hands. While she sat, agitated hands twisted and untwisted on her lap. I quickly learned that she was given to simple declarative sentences spoken in an unnaturally loud voice.

"I'm unhappy."

There was silence. "Go on," I prompted.

"I have of late lost all my mirth."

The phrase seemed oddly formal. Then I remembered it was a quote from *Hamlet*. Patients sometimes use someone else's words so they don't have to use their own. It's a defense, a way of masking feeling. I waited for her to continue. It took a while.

"I used to love my job. Now I hate it. I used to love my husband. Now we're divorced. When I have to see him, I can barely look at him."

"When did the change come?" I asked.

"With the suicide bombings."

The totally unexpected answer stopped me short. Sometimes mood swings from happy to depressed are caused by the death of a parent (Evelyn's father, I learned later, died when she was a child), the loss of a job (clearly not Evelyn's problem), or the effects of a long illness (Evelyn was in excellent health). Suicide bombings, unless one was directly attacked, were, to say the least, an unusual impetus.

She began to weep. "The poor Jews. The poor Jews." She took a deep breath. The tears stopped. "Those *damn* Arabs!"

The swear word seemed out of character, an indication of the rage beneath it. "You're Jewish, then?" I asked.

"With all my heart and soul."

"Your parents, were they as passionate as you?"

"No. They weren't very religious. Neither am I. And they didn't care about Israel. To me it's the one country that matters. The Arabs are out to destroy it."

"And your husband?"

"He *claims* he's Jewish, but he doesn't care about Israel, either. It's one of the reasons I hate him."

She stared at me antagonistically, perhaps because I remained calm in the force of her passion. "Look. I've lost my appetite— for food, for sex, for love, for business. I'm frustrated and unsatisfied. I can't sleep. I know I need psychotherapy. You have a good reputation. Help me."

"So you can find out where the anger and anxiety come from?"

"I want my happiness back." She hung her head. "I go to the movies. I go shopping. I go to bed. And I think about how much I hate the Arabs. I hate the U.N. I know they've done good, but they're dominated by anti-Semites. Every vote goes against Israel. I know I'm overreacting. I know I should care about something else. But those damn Arabs. How can they kill Jewish babies? How *can* I care about anything else?"

We tried conventional psychotherapy, exploring her childhood in this life, but the causes of her anger and her anxiety did not seem to reside there. She agreed to a regression.

"Go back to the time and place where your anger first began," I instructed her when she was in a deep hypnotic state. This was as far as I would lead her. She would pick wherever and whenever that was.

"It's World War Two," she said in a deep masculine voice, sitting up straight with an expression of disbelief. "I'm a Nazi officer, a member of the SS. I have a good job. It is to supervise the loading of Jews into the cattle cars that will take them to Dachau. There they will die. If any of them tries to escape, I shoot them. I don't like to do that. It's not that I care that the vermin dies. It's that I hate to lose a bullet. Bullets are expensive. We've been told to save ammunition whenever possible." Her cold-blooded recitation was belied by the horror in her tone and a slight trembling that possessed her body. As a German she might have felt nothing for the people she killed; as Evelyn, remembering, she was in agony.

I've discovered that the surest way to be reincarnated into a particular group of people, defined by religion, race, nationality, or culture, is to hate those people in a previous life, to be prejudiced or violent against that group. It did not surprise me that Evelyn had been a Nazi. Her intense pro-Israel stance in this life was a compensation for her anti-Semitism in her German one. But she had overcompensated. The hatred she had felt for the Jews had been transformed into an equal hatred for Arabs. No wonder she felt anxious, frustrated, and depressed. She had not moved very far on her journey toward health.

Evelyn went to another part of her German life. The allied army had entered Poland, and she had been killed at the front during a fierce battle. In her life review, after the death in that life, she felt remorse and enormous guilt, but she still needed to return now to confirm that she had learned her lesson and to make up to those she had hurt in her German life.

We are all souls, all part of the One, all the same, whether we are Germans or Jews, Christians or Arabs. But apparently Evelyn had not learned this lesson. Her hatred had not disappeared.

"I want to try an experiment," I told her after I had brought her back to the present. "Are you game for it?" She eagerly agreed.

She made herself comfortable; her hands stopped their anxious play. She looked at me expectantly.

"I believe that we are capable of influencing our future lives by what we do in this one," I said. "Right now you are influencing your future life by your anger toward Arabs, just as you influenced the other one by your hatred of Jews. Now I want to progress you to your next probable life, your life if you stay on your present course and are Evelyn unchanged from the person who came to me for help."

I put her in a deep hypnotic state and directed her to a future life that would have connections to the German soldier's life and to her present life's anti-Arab bias. Her eyes were closed, but it was clear that what they were seeing was vivid. "I'm a Muslim girl. An Arab. A teenager. I'm in a hut made of tin, like the Bedouins use. I've lived there all my life."

"Where is this hut?" I asked.

She frowned. "In the Palestinian territories or in Jordan. It's not clear which. The boundaries have changed."

"When did they change?"

"They are always changing. But everything else is the same. The war with the Jews goes on. Whenever there is a period of peace, the radicals destroy it. It means we are poor. We will always be poor." Her voice grew harsh. "It's the Jews' fault. They are rich, but they don't help us. We are their victims."

I asked her to go forward in her Arab life, but she died soon after "of an illness" and could add nothing further. Instead, she had a brief glimpse of the life after that one. She was a Christian man living in East Africa, angry at the rapidly growing Hindu population in his part of the world. (It's amazing, I thought. Prejudice never ends.) In her life review she recognized that there were and would always be people to hate, but now at last there was an epiphany. "Compassion and love are the antidotes to hatred and rage," she said, her voice full of wonder. "Violence only perpetuates the suffering."

When I brought her back to the present, we discussed what she had learned. She knew she had to alter her assumptions about other peoples and cultures. She needed to replace hatred with understanding. These concepts are easy to understand in the brain, but not easy to assimilate as a way of behavior.

"It took you two possible lifetimes to come to this recognition," I pointed out. "But what if you could speed the change now that you understand the concept in the present? What would your future lives look like then?"

In our next session I progressed Evelyn to a future life that connected the German soldier's life and her present anger. "This time, though, you have to let go of all prejudice in your current life. You see all souls and people as equal, connected to each other by the spiritual energy of love."

A calm came over her. Apparently, her future life changed completely. She did not find Arab or East African lifetimes but instead: "I'm the manager of a hotel in Hawaii. It's a spa as well. A beautiful hotel and spa. There are flowers everywhere. The guests come from all over the world. From different countries and cultures. They come to find recuperative energy. It's easy to find it because the spa is so well managed and its setting is so splendid." She smiled at the vision. "I'm blessed. I get to enjoy the hotel all year round."

It is, of course, a nice fantasy to imagine yourself as the manager of a great spa in a gorgeous setting surrounded by the smell of hibiscus. What Evelyn saw in this voyage into the future might indeed have been fantasy, projection, or wishful thinking. When I regress someone, it's sometimes difficult to separate actual memory from metaphor, imagination, or symbol. In visualized past lives, however, if a person is speaking a foreign language he or she never learned in this one, that is a sign of authenticity. So is accurate historical detail. If the memory brings up intense emotion, that is also a sign. But while intense emotion often accompanies progressions, validation is much more difficult. I operate on the assumption that even though a progression can't be checked out, it is still a powerful healing device. Yes, metaphor and fantasy are possible, but healing is the important part. In regression and progression, symptoms disappear, illnesses get better, and anxiety, depression, and fear are relieved.

No one has figured out a way to confirm that the imagined future is really going to happen. Those few who have joined me in this field are inevitably faced with that ambiguity. If a patient is progressed to a future time in his present life, you can confirm it when the vision comes true. But even then it is possible for a patient who has seen her future to veer her life in that direction. Just because a vision is a fantasy doesn't mean you can't make it come true.

People sit in front of me with their eyes closed. Whatever comes into their minds, whether metaphor, imagination, symbol, fantasy, or actual memory, is all grist for the healing mill. This is the foundation of psychoanalysis, and it is the foundation of the work I do, though the scope of my work is broader in that it takes in the distant past and the future.

From my healer's perspective, it does not matter whether Evelyn's visions of what was past and what is to come are real. It is probable that her German life was real, for it was accompanied by intense emotion. And I know that her visions of her future lives influenced her in a powerful way because they said to her: If you don't change, you're just going to be repeating this destructive cycle of aggressor and victim, but if you do change, you can break the cycle. Her different visions of the future taught her that she had the free will to shape the future and that the time to start exercising that free will was now.

Evelyn decided not to wait until her next life to bring healing recuperation to herself and others. A few months after our final session, she left her firm and opened a bed-and-breakfast in Vermont. She regularly practices yoga and meditation. Outwardly and inwardly—profoundly—she has let go of her anger and her prejudices. Her progressions enabled her to attain the happiness she came to me to find. And in her I found a model for the power of progression and further confidence to use it as a therapeutic tool.

Victoria and Evelyn probably could not have taken their journeys without a therapist to guide them. While it is difficult to practice regression and progression alone, in my workshops I teach healing exercises that can be used at home even when there is no therapist around. I have also made some regression CDs that can be used to aid the process. They can be used to alleviate physical or emotional problems. For any of them to be effective, you must be in a state of deep relaxation.

Many therapists tell you in their books how to relax; whatever works for you is fine. In short form, my method is this: Find a place where you can be alone and will not be interrupted—your bedroom or den, say. Close your eyes. Focus first on your breath, imagining that with each exhalation you are ridding yourself of all the tensions and stresses in your body and that each time you inhale you are breathing in beautiful energy. Then concentrate on the different areas of your body. Relax the muscles of your face, your jaw, your neck, and shoulders. Go on to your back, abdomen, stomach, and legs. Your breathing is regular, relaxed; inhale energy, exhale tension. Next, after relaxing all your muscles, visualize a beautiful light above your head, a healing light that is flowing into your body from the top of your head and down to the tips of your toes, growing warmer and more healing as it descends. When I am leading the exercise, I count backwards at this point from ten to one, but you don't have to do that if you are alone.

Dialogue with Illness[*]

Pick one—and only one—symptom, mental or physical, that you would like to understand and, by understanding, heal. It could be the arthritis in your joints, your fear of heights, or your shyness when you meet a stranger. Notice the first thoughts or feelings or impressions that come into your mind. Do this spontaneously, without editing; these should be your first thoughts, no matter how silly or trivial they might seem. Get in touch with that part of your body or mind that is troubling you. Try to make the symptom worse at first, experiencing it as fully as you can, and observe how you did that. Then, *switch places with the symptom;* you are the symptom, the symptom is you. This is so you can be most fully aware of the symptom. It knows where it is lo-

[*]I have adapted this exercise from similar ones taught by Elizabeth Stratton and others that are used by gestalt therapists.

cated and how it affects the body or mind. Next, have the you that is outside the symptom ask the symptom a series of questions.

+ How have you affected my life?
+ What are you going to do with my body/mind now that you're in it?
+ How have you affected my relationships?
+ Do you help convey something I can't convey without you, some message or some information?
+ Do you protect me from anyone or anything?

This last is the key question, for people often use illnesses to avoid confronting the issues that lie behind them—a form of denial. Let's say, for example, that you are experiencing sharp pains in your neck. The exercise will let you locate exactly who or what that pain in the neck is—your boss, your mother-in-law, a way of holding your head so you don't have to look somebody directly in the eye.

In workshops I ask the questions, so the illness is free to concentrate on its host. If you are doing the exercise at home, prerecord the questions, leaving intervals on the tape long enough for mindful, considered answers. Or you can work with a friend.

This exercise, like the others, is not a panacea; a cancer won't disappear, nor will a mother-in-law. But often the exercise will alleviate symptoms, and occasionally a "miracle" occurs and a cure is effected. We do not know the extent of the mind-body connection—in multiple personalities a rash or fever will disappear when one of the multiples switches to another, or one may be an alcoholic and another intolerant to alcohol—but we know it exists, and these exercises are a means of maximizing the dual force.

Healing Visualization

Here, too, I've adapted the exercise, this time from a number of sources. Again, in workshops I lead the participants, but it can be done at home with the use of a recorder or with a friend or loved one at your side. After a few repetitions you will remember the steps; it is a simple yet often extremely powerful exercise.

With your eyes closed and in a relaxed state, go to an ancient island of healing. The island is beautiful, and the weather itself is a balm. There is no more relaxing place in the world. Embedded in the floor of the ocean, a short way out from the beach, are some very large and powerful crystals that impart a strong healing energy to the water. Step into the water, going only as far as is comfortable; the sea is warm and calm. You'll feel a tingling on your skin. This is the supercharged energy of the crystals absorbed by you through the water that touches your body. Direct the energy to the part of your body that needs healing. It need not be one place; perhaps your entire being is crying out for health. Stay in the water for some time, feeling relaxed and letting the energy work on you in its benevolent way.

Now visualize several tame and loving dolphins swimming up to you, attracted by your calmness and the beauty inside you. Dolphins are master diagnosticians and healers; they add their energy to the energy of the crystals. By this time you can swim as well as the dolphins because the water is so supercharged with energy. Together you play in the water, touching each other, diving, and coming up to breathe the beneficent air. You are so entranced by your newfound friends that you forget the original purpose of the swim, which is to heal, but all the while your body is absorbing the healing energy from the crystals and the dolphins.

When you are ready, leave the water and go back to the beach. You are comforted by the knowledge that you can return as many times as you wish. The sand feels good under your feet. So special is the water that immediately you are dry. Feeling content, happy, and *well,* you sit quietly for a time experiencing the warmth of the sun and the caress of the breezes. Then you allow yourself to emerge from the visualization, from this soft dream, knowing that you can always go back and that the healing will continue even after you are awake.

Regression Visualization

In a relaxed state and with your eyes closed, imagine a spiritual being, someone who is very wise. The spirit can be a relative or a beloved friend who has passed over, or it can be a stranger whom you nevertheless trust and love as soon as there is contact between you. The essential factor is that this person loves you unconditionally. You feel totally safe.

Follow your spirit guide to a beautiful ancient temple of healing and memories. It sits high on a hill surrounded by white clouds. To reach the entrance you climb up beautiful marble steps. When you reach the top, the great doors swing open, and you follow the spirit inside where there are fountains, marble benches, and walls inlaid with scenes of nature at its most abundant. There are others in the room, voyagers like yourself with their own spirit guides; all are relaxed, enchanted.

The spirit leads you to a private room, as elaborate in design as the first but bare of furniture save for a couch set directly in the center of the floor. You lie on it, realizing you have never been so comfortable. Above the couch are suspended crystals of different sizes, shapes, and colors. Under your direction the spiritual being arranges the crystals in such a way that light of the perfect color—green, yellow, blue, and gold—goes like a laser beam to that part of the body or the emotional body, the mind, most in need of healing. The light changes; the crystals have broken it into the colors of the rainbow, all of which you absorb as part of your healing. The spirit directs you to look at one wall of the room, and to your amazement it is blank like a movie screen.

In group sessions I count slowly backward from ten to one and tell the attendees that images of their past lives will appear. In your home you will have to pause before the images take shape. You don't have to go into that past life—there may be more than one—but simply imagine it. The life may appear as a series of photographs, or it may come like a movie. Maybe one scene will keep repeating. It doesn't matter; whatever you see is fine. And all the while you are looking at the screen, your body is absorbing the healing energy beamed from the crystals. The healing is taking place not only in this life but in the past where the wound may have originated. If you see a direct connection between past life roots and present-day symptoms, the healing becomes more pronounced. But even if you don't draw a connection, as often happens, the healing remains powerful. You, the spirit, the temple, the crystals, and the light are working in concert to heal; all are powerful.

Healing Duets: Psychometry

In workshops and seminars I have the people in the audience break up into groups of two, preferably strangers to each other. Each is asked to pick an object in his or her possession to hand to the partner, something small like a bunch of keys, a bracelet, glasses, a necklace, or a ring. The partners exchange objects, and then I have them go into the relaxed state common to all the exercises. "You will receive an impression about the person whose object you hold," I tell them. "It may strike you as strange. It may seem as if the impression has nothing to do with the man or woman you're facing. But no matter how silly or unusual or weird the thought, remember it and then share it with your partner. After all, what seems bizarre to you might have deep significance for him or her."

This is far more than a parlor trick, though it can be great fun. There is a diagnostic component. About one-third of the audience at a workshop I gave in Mexico City picked up a physical symptom of their partner, and participants may be able to discover often forgotten but significant childhood episodes in their partners' lives. For example, at a class I taught at Florida International University in Miami, one young man, who had not met his female partner until that moment, completely and accurately described her tenth birthday party, the one where she was humiliated by her older sister. There was another young man who had been shot in the left forearm while trying to flee a thug attempting to rob him. He wore a long-sleeved shirt, buttoned at the wrist, so his partner, a woman, couldn't have seen the scar. Yet when she held his car keys, she felt a sharp pain in her own left forearm. Some described others' past lives; many described the house where the partner grew up as a child.

At the end of my Mexican workshop I had five people take the microphone to share with the group what they had undergone. Four of them had mediumistic experiences! They received messages from their partners' deceased loved ones, all of them recognized by their partners whom they had never met until that moment. Some were able to describe what the dead person looked like. One told of a six-year-old girl whom he saw walking backward, which to him meant that the girl had died. The girl was saying, "I'm fine. I'm okay. You don't have to grieve so much. I love you." His partner, a woman, started to weep. She had lost her six-year-old daughter a few months before.

This exercise can be done at home, though it is most effective if you do it with someone you know casually or have only recently met. While you are healing your partner by delivering a message or picking up a physical or emotional symptom—anxiety, depression, sadness—an extraordinary connection quickly develops, and there is a feedback effect that is as powerful for you as it is for your partner.

Long-Distance Healing

In a relaxed state, with your eyes closed, visualize loved ones who may be physically sick or emotionally troubled. By sending them healing light, healing energy, your prayers (you don't have to believe in any formal religion), and your love, you can actually affect their recovery—as far out as this sounds. Scientific evidence backs my statement. Dr. Larry Dossey's book, *Reinventing Medicine,* points to a number of studies which show that among heart patients, those who were prayed for from afar had better clinical outcomes than those receiving medical therapy alone. A double-blind study of advanced AIDS patients found that even when they did not know they were being prayed for, they experienced fewer and less severe AIDS-related illnesses.

My own technique is to take one person in a workshop of, say, eighty people and put him or her in the middle of a circle formed by the rest of the attendees. I ask them to project healing energy into that person, silently but with all their spiritual force.

I have said that the healing exercises are most effective when directed toward one specific ailment. With Victoria it was the cancer in her back. With Evelyn it was the anxiety that consumed her night and day. Most people have a susceptible organ or part of their body that seems to be the first affected under conditions of stress or incipient disease. It may be the throat and respiratory system, the back, the skin, the heart, and so on.

In Michelle, another remarkable woman, the area was the knees. She remembered her left knee being lacerated by a submerged rock when as a child she went into the water at the beach near her home. When she was under stress as an adult, she often felt migratory stabbing pains in both knees but more so on the left. Anxiety, she told me, left her "weak-kneed." She occasionally experienced swelling and edema, particularly after an athletic injury in college that required minor surgery on her left knee; arthroscopic surgery was needed later. By the time I met her, CAT scans and X-rays showed cartilage loss. She could not fully extend her left leg because of the damage, and by now she walked with a slight limp. She was aware, though, that the damage was emotional as well as physical, which is why she came to see me.

Her first regression brought her back briefly to the rural Midwest of nineteenth-century America. Her name was Emma, and in middle age she had been run down by a horse-drawn wagon. The accident shattered her left knee and shin and also badly damaged her right knee. A subsequent infection left her permanently disabled. In a glimpse of another life, Michelle saw herself in medieval Japan as a male soldier whose left knee was pierced by an arrow.

Both regressions explained her present knee troubles but did not get to the origin of the karmic lesson, so we kept going and soon reached North Africa in pre-Roman times. Michelle was once again a man, this time a warden at a particularly brutal prison who took special delight in destroying the legs of the prisoners so they could not escape. Sometimes he would hamstring a prisoner with a sword or knife; sometimes he smashed their knees with a hammer or a rock. He broke femurs, drove spikes through knees, and severed Achilles' tendons. Many of his captives died from the infections of their wounds, but he reveled in their misery. His superiors took a vicarious delight in dispatching prisoners to his care, and he was well rewarded for his violence, living in considerable luxury amid the squalor of the place.

Michelle was disturbed by this regression, and it took another session before she achieved complete integration and understanding. Eventually she realized that we have all passed through barbaric lives and that she, like the rest of us, should feel no shame or guilt for what we did millennia in the past. Our journey is upward. We have all evolved through lifetimes of violence and cruelty. The Old Testament says that the sins of the father are visited on the children into the third and fourth generation, that we are being affected negatively by what our fathers did before us. But *we* are our fathers, just as we will be our children. The sins of our own pasts will haunt our presents until we can understand them and earn absolution. The sins of this lifetime will darken our futures, but as we acted wisely in the past, so our presents are made lighter. If we act humanely now, we will bring our future selves closer to the One.

Michelle was able to see why her knees and legs were so painful in her present life. She had paid a heavy price for her past behaviors, but now, she recognized, she could be freed. During a deep trance state she went back again to that North African life, but this time instead of inflicting pain, she was the one who felt it, and she asked for forgiveness and grace. She could not change the facts and details of that life, but she could alter her reactions to those events on a *spiritual* level. This process of going back is called *reframing*. It doesn't change the facts, but it changes how you react to the facts. Michelle sent thoughts of light and healing to the prisoners or, rather, to their higher selves, their souls. And she was able to forgive herself. "I know how to break the cycle," she said through tears of gratitude. "Through love and compassion."

She began to get better. The inflammation in her knees receded. She developed full range of motion in her legs, and radiographic examination showed both knees completely healed. Her stress-related weak-kneed state was erased. She was free to explore and understand other more sophisticated lessons of compassion and empathy. She supported organizations that advocate for the abolition of land mines (which often cause crippling leg injuries) and those that fight against cruelty to animals. She has received grace.

Michelle did not want to go into the future, but I know what it will be. In this life she will continue her humanitarian work, and with each act she will progress toward a better state in her next lifetime and the lifetimes to come. In those lives she will be free of the physical problems with her legs, for she has expiated her North African sins. I don't know what her professions will be or whom she will meet and love, but she will perform and love with charity and compassion.

CHAPTER 4

Samantha and Max:
Empathy

A FEW DAYS before I began this chapter, my wife Carole's uncle lay dying of cancer in a Miami hospital. She and he were very close, and this was an ordeal for her. I was close to him, too, though not nearly to the degree Carole was, so when I visited his hospital room, my focus was less on him than on her and on his children gathered at his bedside. (His wife had passed away many years earlier.) I could feel their sadness, their pain, and their grief. This was empathy on my part, an emotion that grows as we get older, for the degree to which we empathize is influenced by undergoing similar situations in our own lives. I had lost both a child and my father and thus knew the pain of confronting the death of a loved one. It was not difficult for me to experience the emotions of the people in that room; I know what grief feels like, and I felt a strong kinship with them all even though I had met the children only a few times over the years. I was able to reach out to them, and they could accept my words of comfort, knowing they were genuine. They empathized with me as well.

Around the same time an earthquake in Iran killed some forty thousand people and left hundreds of thousands wounded, torn from their families, and without homes. There were horrific scenes on television of people digging out the wounded and the dead. I watched in horror. A different kind of empathy was at work here, more global and probably not as painful as the emotions I felt in that hospital room. If there had been no pictures of the earthquake's aftermath, I might have felt very little; it was the *individuality* of tragedy, along with the immediacy of the pictures, that made it so painful.

My empathy went as much to the rescuers as to the victims, and I found myself thinking that this world is such a difficult place. Here we have illness, disease, earthquakes, typhoons, floods, all the calamities of nature, and yet we add war, violence, and murder. Like many nations the United States immediately pledged relief aid in the form of food, medicine, and manpower. Yet, we were assured, Iran was still part of the axis of evil, and it was right to hate their leaders. If it could be claimed they were a threat to us, we would go to war.

Madness!

Empathy is the ability to put yourself in someone else's place—to feel their feelings, to be in their situation, to see through their eyes. If we are capable of empathy, we can bond with those who are suffering, rejoice in another's love, feel pleasure at someone else's triumph, and understand a friend's anger and a stranger's grief. It is a trait that, when mastered and correctly used, can help bring us further toward the future. Those lacking empathy cannot spiritually evolve.

The core principle underlying empathy is that we are all connected. I began to understand it during the height of the Cold War when I saw a movie about a Russian soldier. I knew I was supposed to hate him, but as he went through his daily ritual— shaving, having breakfast, going into the field for training—I remember thinking, "This soldier is only a few years older than I. He may have a wife and children who love him. Perhaps he is being forced to fight for political ideas that are those of his leaders but with which he disagrees. I've been told he's my enemy, but if I looked into his eyes, wouldn't I see myself? Aren't I being told to hate myself?"

That Russian soldier of yesterday and the Arab soldier of today are the same as you are, for they both have souls and you have a soul, and all souls are one. In our past lifetimes we have changed races, sexes, economic circumstances, living conditions, and religions. We will change them in the future as well. So if we hate or if we fight or if we kill, we are hating and fighting and killing ourselves.

Empathy teaches this lesson; it is one of the feelings we are put on Earth to learn, a key aspect of our preparation for immortality. It is a difficult lesson in that we must experience it not only in our mind but in our physical bodies, and in the mind and body we have pain, dark emotions, difficult relationships, enemies, loss, and grief. We thus tend to forget others and concentrate on ourselves. But we also have love, beauty, music, art, dance, nature, and air, and we long to share them. We cannot transform negativity into the positive without empathy, and we cannot truly understand empathy without experiencing it in our present life, in our past, and in our future.

Samantha experienced it. It literally changed her forever.

She was a frail girl, weighing less than a hundred pounds, and she sat in my office on a February morning with her shoulders hunched and her hands clasped firmly on her stomach, as though to hold in pain. Her clothes were simple: jeans, sweater, sneakers with ankle socks, and no jewelry, not even a watch. She might just be entering high school, I thought, though I knew from my introductory questions, to which she gave subdued, barely audible answers, that she was in fact nineteen and a college freshman. Her parents had sent her to me because she was suffering from severe anxiety and low-grade depression.

"I can't sleep," she said in a voice so soft I had to strain to hear it. Indeed, her eyes were watery and bloodshot.

"Do you know why?" I asked.

"I'm worried I'm going to fail my courses."

"All of them?"

"No. Just math and chemistry."

"Why not take different subjects?" I winced. It was a stupid question. Those were the courses she had selected. And, indeed, she bristled.

"They're prerequisites."

"For med school?" I ought to know. They had been the focus of my college years.

"Yes. And I *creamed* the math SAT."

"So you want to be a doctor?" I sounded banal, I knew, but I was searching for a point of entry, something that would rouse her from the defeated young woman sitting opposite me.

At last she raised her head and met my eyes. "More than anything. It's what I'm *going* to be."

"But you can't get into med school unless you pass math and chemistry."

She nodded. Her eyes kept contact. I had identified her problem, and this very fact had given her a little hope. "Tell me. Did you have trouble with your math and science courses in high school?"

"A little." She paused. "No, a lot, though you wouldn't know it from the SATs."

I wondered if she'd experienced too much parental pressure. "Do your mom and dad want you to be a doctor?"

"They want whatever I want. They've been *wonderful*. Supportive, kind, loving—I couldn't have better parents. They got me a tutor to help me with my studies. But she doesn't do much good. I just look at the numbers and the formulas, and I go blank."

She spoke with such fervor, such passion, that for the first time I saw what an extraordinary young woman Samantha was.

The pressure did not seem to be parental but internal. I was sure that her sense of defeat was not so ingrained that it couldn't be overcome.

"And now you feel you're letting them down."

"Yes, and it makes me miserable. I'm letting my brother down, too. Sean. He's eleven and has a weak heart, and he has to be careful. But it's really *myself* I'm letting down most of all. Dr. Weiss, I go into a classroom to take a test, even the simplest quiz, and before I sit down, I start trembling and sweating, and I begin to panic and want to run away. Once, I actually did. Just ran out of that room and back to my dorm and lay on the bed and sobbed."

"What happened?"

"Oh, I told them I was sick, and they let me take the quiz again. They'll let me take my midterms again, too—the ones I failed last month, the ones I'll fail again. Fail and fail and fail and fail."

She broke down, weeping with an anguish born of months of despair. I let her cry—it would have been futile to try to stop her—but at last the tears ceased, and, to my amazement, she managed a wan and endearing smile. "I'm a mess," she said. "My whole life's down the tubes. Fix me."

I knew we would have to find the source of her block. Perhaps it lay in a different life. I thought of regressing her to find out, but I wanted to learn more before we began.

"What about your grades in other courses?"

"Straight A's. I'm not dumb."

No, I didn't think so. "Then let's say, just hypothetically, you couldn't pass math and chemistry and had to choose a different future. Would that be so terrible?"

"It would be impossible," she said calmly.

"Not really. You're still young. There are a million paths open to you."

"Don't you understand?" she asked. "There's only the one."

I didn't understand. "Why?"

"Because I've seen my future. I've seen it in my dreams."

Electricity. "You've *seen* it?"

If she shared my excitement, she did not show it. "Yes. But I don't get how it will happen—not if I can't pass my exams."

"How do you know the dream is really about your future, that what you see will happen?"

"Because when I've dreamt about the future before, it comes true." Sadness crept back into her voice. "Only this time it *can't* happen. Something is stopping it."

She was going too fast. "Backtrack a second," I said. "Give me an example of a dream that came true."

"I had a dream that my friend Diana would get hurt in a car crash. Two weeks later she did, just like I saw it. Another car hit hers when she stopped at an intersection." She shuddered. "Creepy."

She described other precognitive dreams—a mountain climbing accident and the early arrival home of her father from a business trip.

Many people have precognitive dreams, visions of events about to happen; I had encountered them several times before. But with Samantha, many of her future dreams were more textured, more vivid, and more elaborate. She was seeing not an incident but a detailed later life.

"I'm in med school. It's a great university, so there are scores of other students. It's graduation day. June. We're seated on a stage, and the dean is handing out diplomas. There's a huge audience, the women in frilly, flowery dresses, so maybe the university is in the South. Flags are waving in the hot breeze. My parents are in the first row, and I can see them beaming at me, proud of me as I am of myself. The dean calls my name. I have graduated, he announces, with the highest honors. I walk to the lectern where he is standing, and he hands me my diploma, which is rolled up and tied with a ribbon. The audience begins to cheer, not only my parents but all of them. The other students are cheering, too, and I'm so happy I could burst. I go back to my seat, untie the ribbon, and open the diploma. It is the most beautiful thing I've ever seen. My name is printed in red like a neon sign and—"

She started to cry, tears as large as drops from a faucet. "It's not going to happen. Maybe I should take a leave of absence, leave school before I fail a course so it won't be on my record. Maybe I should *marry* a doctor."

"Maybe you won't have to. Maybe we can find out where that block is coming from." My words did little to encourage her. Her head was bowed once more, and her hands clasped at her stomach. "Any other dreams?" I asked.

"It's a few years later. I'm a doctor now, walking down a hospital corridor, going from one patient's room to another. The patients are children—I'm a *pediatrician!* It's what I always wanted to be. I love kids, and it's obvious they like me, for every one of them, even the littlest and sickest, with tubes coming from their noses and arms, are glad to see me. I'm thrilled that I have the expertise to help them. One little boy takes my hand. I sit by his bedside until he falls asleep."

The dreams could be anything: fantasies, precognitive dreams, dreams of the future, or metaphors having nothing to do with medicine at all. But they were certainly real to Samantha, and she grew sadder when she related the second one, for she felt the barrier between her future and present—the unscalable mountain of math and chemistry—stood before her. She could see no way to bridge it.

We scheduled several additional sessions quickly because she had to determine whether to stay in school, which was impossible if she couldn't get through her exams. I know that doctors are supposed to be objective, but I felt a special affinity for Samantha. She reminded me of my own daughter, Amy, who had her own dreams, her own bright future.

Samantha came back two days later. When she was in a deep hypnotic trance, I instructed her to proceed along the pathway of her optimal future. Unerringly, the medical school graduation and the proud pediatrician images reappeared, this time in even more detail, from the green trim of her academic robe to the antiseptic smell of the hospital corridors. "This is my future," she insisted confidently when I asked her to explore alternatives in her current life. She would not be dissuaded, math and chemistry notwithstanding. The session did not change her sense of frustration, but it did seem to motivate her to stay in school and go on with her therapy. There was more hope somehow and her strong sense that her dreams of the future would be realized. Urgency and fear were still present, but now she became more patient, and there was a resolute will to progress. "I'll make it," she kept repeating.

If she believed, so did I.

In the next session it was from a deep level that I led her into a past life. "I see a man," Samantha said. "He's not me, and yet he is me. He's an architect, and his job is to design buildings for the agora—for kings. He's a master at spatial relations, at geometric designs. But these buildings are special. This is the most important commission he has ever received. They're complicated designs and he's worried that he won't get them right, but the computations are difficult and the answers don't come to him. Oh, I'm sorry for him—for me! He's a fine musician and plays a flute at night to ease his spirits, but tonight the music does him no good. He's straining and struggling, but the answers just won't come. Poor man. If he can't—"

She stopped in mid-sentence, her expression one of puzzlement. Her eyes remained closed. "Wait a minute. I'm not in Greece anymore but in Rome. It's a few hundred years later. There's another man. A civil engineer. Again he's me and not me. He designs buildings, bridges, roadways, aqueducts. He knows the composition and capabilities of the materials he uses, knows how to make sure that what he builds will last forever. He's an expert mathematician as well. He's considered the best. He *is* the best. I'm so happy for him, I could cry."

* * *

In early regressions it is not unusual for one life to "interrupt" another, so I wasn't surprised by Samantha's sudden leap from Greek times to Roman. And taken by themselves, the two past lives were not remarkable. There were no powerful spiritual insights, no tragedies, traumas, or catastrophes that might have led us to an understanding of her present blockage. Yet the dual regression was nevertheless immensely important because Samantha was able to connect emotionally and viscerally with the struggling Greek architect and the civil engineer. She *empathized* with them. She could well understand the frustration of the architect, and she felt the triumph of the engineer because she had known the same feelings in her dreams of the future. In effect, she was empathizing with herself. She knew she was architect and engineer, and that was enough for her to let go of her present symptom. In a sense she already possessed a powerful mathematic and problem-solving ability, learned in the past.

I could see immediately that her new perception of herself was carried over from the regression experience. She became much more confident in speech and bearing. Her self-image had been transformed. The block would soon be gone, I mused, and indeed this shift in her consciousness manifested itself almost immediately in an "aha" comprehension of the mathematical and chemical concepts that had been eluding her.

With the continued help of her tutor, Samantha's math and science grades began improving as early as the next round of tests, and the positive reinforcement from her improved scores increased her confidence even more. I continued to see her for almost a year, then terminated therapy, convinced that she would achieve the promise of her dreams. At the end of her senior year in college she came to see me.

"I did it!" she exclaimed.

I knew what she meant but let her explain. "Did what?"

"Got into med school."

"Good for you!" I said, deeply gratified. "Where?"

Her eyes twinkled, and she gave me an impish grin. "You see, Dr. Weiss, my dreams of the future aren't always infallible. The school isn't in the South. I'm going to Cornell."

Samantha, a budding doctor, showed empathy for herself in the past and therefore could move toward her future. Max, an experienced doctor, showed his empathy for others in the past and therefore could *see* his future and transform his present.

When I met him initially, he was, to put it bluntly, obnoxious (even doctors make snap judgments at first meetings), and I wasn't the only one who couldn't stand him. He was a doctor at a neighboring hospital, and many of his patients and colleagues felt the same way. Indeed, it was one of his colleagues, Betsy Prager, a psychologist, who sent him to me for treatment. Better my office than hers was her attitude. She said the hospital staff had pretty much ordered him into therapy.

He arrived like a summer squall, high winds and high heat, pacing in front of my desk in a state of advanced anxiety. "I shouldn't be here," he announced. "No need for it. Those bastards who run the hospital think I should be toned down. I think they should be fired. They're not letting me do my job."

He was a tall man of thirty-eight with jowly red face, unkempt thinning brown hair, and eyes flashing fire. Dressed in tan slacks and a Hawaiian shirt, he looked more like a bartender than a physician.

"Jesus!" he went on. "This night nurse. Typical woman. One of my patients—great guy, a true prince, heroic, super family—has meningitis. Calls for her. He's vomiting. She wouldn't get off the phone. I screamed at her to stop talking. She claimed her son was sick. Fat chance. And when she hung up, I let her have it, threatened to beat her brains out."

"When was this?"

"Last week. The bitch reported me. I guess that's why Dr. Prager called you."

"What time did you threaten her?" I asked quietly.

"Midnight. Maybe after."

"What were you doing at the hospital so late?"

"My job. Looking after my patients."

"Dr. Prager says you're often late and always tired. She tells me you take on duties a resident or intern could handle."

"Yeah, if they didn't have brains in their ass instead of their heads." He put his hands on my desk and leaned toward me confidentially. "You know how it is. You can't trust 'em. I tell them what to do down to the smallest detail, and they always seem to screw it up. Leave 'em with a patient, kiss off the patient."

When I worked at Mount Sinai, almost all the residents and interns were dedicated and competent, eager to learn and to help. Once I got to know them, I trusted them up to the limits of their knowledge. How different could his hospital be? "Don't you get exhausted working at that pace?"

"Sometimes," he acknowledged, sitting down at last. He seemed to welcome the chair, for he visibly relaxed, though one foot jiggled against the floor. Then his agitation flared again. "Of course I get tired. Who wouldn't? If you knew the extent of incompetence I see every day, it'd blow your mind. Wrong doses. Wrong diagnoses. Wrong diets. Incivility, back talk, filth on the floors, incorrect charts . . ." He trailed off like a dying engine.

"Endangering your patients?" I prompted.

The engine refired. "You bet, endangering them! Sometimes"—he leaned toward me again, and his voice dropped to a whisper—"they die."

Yes, some patients die. Maybe the man with meningitis would die. But very few deaths can be ascribed to mistreatment at the hospital or medical malpractice. Cancer kills. Viruses kill. Automobile accidents kill. "But that's inevitable," I said.

"Not with my patients."

This was said so positively and with such arrogance that I recoiled. "Surely some of them," I said. "The cancer patients. The aged. The stroke victims."

A strange thing happened: His eyes filled with tears. "True. And every time it happens, I want to kill myself. I love my patients, every one of them, and when one of them dies, I die with them. It rips me up inside."

"You shouldn't—" I started but then gave up trying to contradict or console him.

"You know who I get angriest at?" He sobbed. "Me."

We went on in this vein for the rest of the session. It turned out that he was obsessive-compulsive about every detail of his patients' medical care, though not in other aspects of his life. I guessed that his patients liked his attention at first but then some of them resented it, for they must have sensed the anxiety attached to his obsessiveness. He was overly involved with his patients emotionally as well. Again, the bonding was probably welcomed at the start, before his hovering made them nervous.

Max suffered alongside his patients. His anxiety about them would develop into despair and remorse if they failed to recuperate. Each setback was his fault, each death unforgivable. As we got to know each other, he told me he prescribed antidepressant medicines for himself when the emotional pain became too great. He began experiencing chest pains and, terrified, rushed to a cardiologist. The cardiologist could find nothing wrong although he conducted a battery of tests. Still, the pains persisted, often debilitatingly so. Incapable of delegating, especially by phone, Max went to the hospital far more frequently than necessary—"just to make sure everyone was all right," as he put it. But this meant he had little time for his family, and even the hours he spent with them were marred by his mood swings and sudden outbursts of temper. In time I became sorry for him.

"I expect all my patients to get better," Max said flatly. Thus he derived no satisfaction when they did get better. A patient's joy was not matched by his own. Max's was hardly a case of a physician feeling omnipotent and somehow expecting perfection with all his patients. Each time a patient got worse, he felt less sure of himself, less worthy of the title "doctor." His bluster, his verbal attacks, and his rage were all a cover for one underlying fact: He was afraid.

Max's physical and psychological symptoms were dangerous, even life-threatening. After careful probing on both our parts, the causes of his distress did not seem to lie in the present or in his childhood. I explained past life therapy, telling him that whether it was real or could be interpreted as metaphor, symbol, or fantasy was not the point, healing was—and that many of my patients got better. "Would you like to try it?" I asked.

"Hell, no! I'll find out I was an axe murderer."

Unlikely, but I didn't dispute him. "Would you like to go into the future then?"

He brightened. "Sure. It's bound to be better than the present."

Often logical, left-brain patients—doctors and lawyers, for example—find progression easier than regression. They figure it is all imagination anyway. In my practice, though, much more than imagination usually flows forth.

Max's body quickly relaxed, and he went to a deeper level, a welcome respite from his everyday life. It didn't take long for a clear image to arise. He saw himself as a teacher of many healers, a physician of the near future, surrounded by his students in a kind of celestial amphitheater.

"The work is satisfying," he told me. "Most of them are better doctors than I am, but I'm able to go beyond the body to the emotions. I teach them how consciousness separates from the body so we can understand the mechanisms of spiritual healing. You see, consciousness goes in stages. First it hovers over the physical body, reviewing its emotional life and preparing to go higher. Then it leaves the emotional body behind as well, all the while becoming lighter and lighter. In this state I call it the 'mental body.' Finally, it separates from this realm and is free to adjust its natural vibration to the spheres, so it can go to even higher states."

He turned his head toward me with great seriousness, teaching me as well as his students in the future, though in his hypnotized state he was unaware of my actual presence.

"When we understand how the four stages interact and affect each other, clues to psychological and bodily healing on the physical plane can be discovered, analyzed, and applied. This is my area of research, and it will change medicine forever. I call my course The Multidimensional Healing of All Energy Bodies."

His description was so clear and verified the vision of other patients so much that I felt a thrill of recognition. His area of research was mine. "It will change medicine forever," he said. This was my own belief, though usually I leave the thought unsaid. From our earlier sessions I knew that Max had never read any New Age books or spiritual texts—he considered the whole field worthless—so he could not have picked up the ideas from prior reading. A Methodist, he had received standard religious training, but it did not remotely approach the topics and concepts he taught in the future. He had no belief in the metaphysical. It is probable that he had never used such phrases as "spiritual healing" and "mental body" in his life.

"What the hell was that all about?" he asked when I brought him back to the present. He seemed amused rather than awed by his experience.

"Who knows?" I answered. Then I told him merely that the pattern of physician, teacher, and healer was not surprising, given his current profession, and that although I was no expert, his observations seemed to have similarities to certain metaphysical concepts I had heard about over the years.

My thoughts, however, went further. What he experienced was not a fantasy, I believe, but elements of his consciousness constructing an archetype of what he wished to be in his next life.

What he saw tied in to others' near death experiences, but he went further, to a place where he could talk about human consciousness and see it climbing toward the One.

"I want to go back now," he said in our next session, still excited by his journey.

"To past lives?"

"You got it. The future was great. How bad can the past be? Besides, I'm curious."

I reminded him that he had control over the process and that he could always stop or adjust the experience or even move to a different life if he wanted.

Once again he went easily into a trance state, and I led him to the past. To my surprise, given his unpleasant male chauvinism, he was a woman.

"I am young, beautiful, married to a good man. It's—what? The twelfth century, thirteenth century? I live in a small community in Europe, Eastern Europe. I've had many illnesses throughout my life, and maybe that's why I became a healer, though I'm happiest among my animals and plants. When I was pregnant, I had scarlet fever and lost my child. I can't have another. It makes me and my husband very sad.

"When people are sick, they call for me, for they know that when I touch them or if I treat them with my herbs and plants, they get better. Sometimes it seems a miracle. Some of the people accept me and are kind to me and my husband, but most of them, I think, are afraid of me. They think I'm a witch and have supernatural powers. They think I'm weird or crazy. But I'm not. I'd just rather be with animals and plants than with them.

"There's this one man, who lives in a nearby village. He's always shouting at me to go away and warning the neighborhood children not to get near me. But now he needs me, and he comes to fetch me. His wife has delivered a stillborn daughter, a daughter who died just like mine, and now she's delirious and is 'burning up.' I rush with him to his house. His wife is very sick. She's having trouble breathing, and her temperature is high. I place my hands on her abdomen, over her uterus. I feel a familiar energy come from my hands, a burst of healing energy transmitting itself to her. I use the plants and herbs to treat her fever. But it's not going to work—*it's not going to work!*"

Max became agitated in my office. His breathing was fast, and there was anguish in his expression. There was no danger to him in his trance state—there never is in anyone's—but he was obviously empathizing with the young girl and with himself as he recalled these ancient events.

"I'm right," Max said, still in the trance. "I'm too late. The infection has overwhelmed the poor mother's defenses. She dies even as my energy flows into her. No one could have saved her. It is the greatest defeat of my life."

Max's agitation increased. "The woman's husband is furious! He has been drinking throughout the process—I've barely noticed him—and now he's distraught, out of his mind, at the loss of his wife so soon after his baby died. 'You killed her, you devil! You witch!' he screams, and before I can defend myself, he raises a knife and plunges it into my chest. I'm in shock. I can't believe it. There's this sharp pain in my chest. It's as though the knife has reached my heart!"

Max doubled over in pain but just as quickly relaxed. "I'm floating now, and when I look down, I can see my body lying on the floor in that man's cabin. It's calm. There's a golden light in the sky, and it touches me. A healing light."

I brought him back to the present. Max had undergone a lot in that single session. He was not amused now, but he wasn't upset. He was pensive and serious, reflecting on that lifetime centuries ago. It was, he knew, his life; he was that healer. We discussed his feelings then and now, the physical pain, the anxiety, the empathy he felt for the dying mother then and the empathy he felt for the young healer now. The experience was much more emotional than that of the consciousness researcher of the future. But, I pointed out, that researcher had given Max the key to unlock this past life. Now he would be able to use that past life, particularly the empathy he felt for the mother and healer, to guide him in the present.

Over the next weeks the changes in Max were apparent to his family, his colleagues, his patients, and me. His chest pain disappeared now that he knew its root cause. He understood that although he had been killed for failing to heal his patient in his prior life, just as he wanted to "kill himself" when he failed in this one, then and now the patients' deaths were not his fault. He realized that he could use his knowledge and medical expertise to do his best, but that he couldn't always control the outcome. Most patients would do well, but some would not for a variety of reasons beyond his skill. His anxiety about his current patients diminished steadily and eventually disappeared. His rages also vanished. He was no longer unrealistic about his performance or the performance of the staff. He made friends among his colleagues and became closer to his family. And he no longer suffered from the guilt, remorse, or depression that had plagued his life before his voyages to the past and to the future.

Max has kept in touch. His diagnostic and therapeutic skills are, he tells me, "better honed" since his therapy. In our last conversation he admitted that when the other medical staff is not looking, he'll place his hands on the area of the patient's body that needs healing and feel the surge of energy he remembers from centuries ago.

The ability to empathize with past and future versions of themselves liberated both Samantha and Max from the tyranny of their present-day fears. For them and for all of us empathy is the key to forgiveness. When we feel a deep emotional identification with younger versions, even past-life manifestations of ourselves, we can appreciate the circumstances that led to our present symptoms and negative judgments. When we understand our negative impulses and can see where they originated in ourselves, we can let go of them. When we do, self-esteem increases, and we are able to see ourselves more favorably.

Equally, empathy is the key to understanding and forgiving others. Through empathy we can comprehend their fears, their beliefs, and their needs. These will often be identical to our own. We can understand them even if we don't fully share their beliefs. We will know on a deep emotional level where they are coming from in their souls. To hate them is to hate ourselves; to love them is to love ourselves. The only sane course is to let go of hate.

Empathy heals the individual at the same time that it heals the world. It is the sister of compassion and the child of unconditional love.

CHAPTER 5

Hugh and Chitra: Compassion

E MPATHY AND COMPASSION are often used synonymously, but they are really two different elements in the human psyche. True, when you understand another's feelings as your own and are able to put yourself in his or her place, you will almost surely become compassionate toward that person. But you can also be compassionate without empathy. You can feel compassion for someone or even an insect or animal even if you don't recognize the other's feelings in yourself.

In Buddhist teaching you are instructed to be compassionate toward animals and insects because all living creatures have souls; indeed, they may have been humans in their past lives and may be humans again. (I don't find this in my work, but it doesn't mean the concept isn't true. It may simply be that humans don't remember lifetimes as a different species.) Thus, you can be compassionate toward a beetle or a bear without empathizing with it, without putting yourself in the insect's or animal's place.

Compassion comes from the heart, and it is illustrated by being kind and benevolent to all living things. Christ was supremely compassionate; by all accounts so was Mohandas Gandhi. When "your heart goes out to someone," you are being compassionate. The "random acts of kindness" that many speak about—letting someone go ahead of you in a checkout line; relinquishing your subway seat to a pregnant woman; giving food to the homeless—are all examples of compassionate behavior, but only if they come from a genuine impulse to be kind and not because you are "doing the right thing" or expect brownie points in heaven.

Compassion is more instinctual, empathy more intellectual; they come from different places. If you do the "Dialogue with Illness" exercise described in chapter 3 and change places with, say, your abusive father, you don't necessarily have to be compassionate toward him. You may realize: "Wow, my father's father did the same thing to him that he's doing to me. He took the cruel things he learned from his father, from his culture, and from his peers, and transmitted them undigested to me. I empathize with what he felt because I understand those feelings, and I'm going to break the transmission of negative behavior because of what I learned."

That is an intellectual exercise. However, ideally, and even in as extreme a case as an abusive father, as you empathize with your father, you can begin to feel compassion for him. This may be difficult; he may be just as cruel to you as before. But he is an injured human being like yourself, and that realization might allow you a heartfelt response as well as an intellectual one. If you do respond, if you can see beyond your injuries, you'll find that as empathy and compassion merge, they lead you toward the final destination of all the lessons on the route to immortality: spiritual love, unconditional love, love that is pure and everlasting.

"I've heard you're famous for treating people by taking them back to their past lives. Is this true?"

The caller was a man named Hugh, and if I was "famous" in my field, so was he in his. He was a psychic medium whose local television show drew an audience of many thousands, the bulk of them wishing to contact loved ones who had died. I'm not psychic myself except to the extent that all of us are sometimes psychic (the "hunch" that leads to the correct business decision; the "surety" that makes us choose one life path over another), but I know it exists. I admire those like John Edward and James Van Praagh who seem to possess it and use it for healing, and I have long since learned not to denigrate things I do not understand.

"I've had some success regressing patients," I acknowledged. "Does this call concern therapy?"

"Yes. Mine." He gave a nervous high-pitched laugh. "Psychic, heal thyself? I don't seem to be able to do it on my own."

We made an appointment for the following week, and I awaited it eagerly. I had treated other psychic patients before and found them to be uniformly interesting. Their extreme sensitivity and their openness to the concept of past lives made them particularly suited to regression therapy.

Hugh was a slight man, short and thin, looking far less imposing than he did the one time I had watched his program— such is the power of television. His face was ruddy from the continued use of makeup, and his clothes (chinos and black T-shirt) seemed one size too large. He was obviously nervous, for his glances darted around the room like fireflies, and he frequently had to clear his throat before he could get out a sentence, though once he started, he was eloquent.

"What's the trouble?" I asked.

"I'm exhausted. Bone tired. It's not physical, though I don't exercise enough, but mental. I feel as if all the people in the world are after me, wanting me to connect them to those they've lost. And they're so needy, so insistent, so worthy, so legitimately hungry that when I say no, I feel guilty—enormous guilt that weighs a million pounds. I can't get it off my back."

People in the mall or even on the street would ask him for readings or information or messages from the beyond, but it doesn't work like that. It's not as if he can dial up someone's relative, leap to the beyond, and deliver a message on cue. It takes energy, strength, and time to work as he does, and it sapped him. I empathized. The same kind of well-meaning assault has happened to me to some extent; I, too, have been stopped in restaurants or breaks during workshops. But people know regression is a time-consuming process and understand without bitterness that I can't accommodate them. People seemed to think Hugh could access the messages left for them while he was eating dinner. He wanted to help—oh, how he wished he could help every one of them! That he couldn't made him feel worthless, and with each rejected request his anxiety increased.

He was, he told me, both clairvoyant and clairaudient—that is, he had the ability to see things happening before they occurred or at a distance, beyond the view of the human eye, and also hear messages spoken only to himself. Like most psychics, these abilities manifested themselves very early. Many children, for example, have imaginary friends, often simply because they're lonely and crave companionship. In some cases, however, the friends are not imaginary at all. In *Through Time into Healing* I wrote about a young girl whose mother couldn't understand why she showed no grief at the death of her grandmother. "Why should I be sad?" the girl asked. "I was just talking to her. She's sitting in a chair in my room." That the grandmother told the child secrets about the mother's childhood—secrets she could not have discovered on her own—validated the story. Other children, seeing accidents or hearing messages that turn out to be true, have added to the evidence of psychic phenomena.

Usually, a child's psychic powers disappear before he or she reaches the age of six. Occasionally, though, the powers not only remain but grow stronger. This is what happened with Hugh.

"When I was a kid," he said, "the other children thought I was weird. 'That's crazy,' they'd say when I told them I'd seen a dead person who spoke to me or tried to warn them about a message I'd received. Sometimes their families told them not to play with me. They made me *feel* crazy, but that didn't stop the visions or the messages. So what I did was keep them to myself, hide them from everybody. I was different then." He paused and cleared his throat. "And I'm different now."

The low self-esteem he had developed as a child continued into adulthood, and for several sessions we worked on that issue and on others associated with it. But I already knew that we would have to go deeper than just childhood sensitivities. I suggested regression. "That's why I'm here," he said, smiling.

Hugh easily entered the trance state (he had been practicing, in a way, since he was a little boy). "I see flying vehicles," he began. "Not exactly planes, but more like cars that can fly, powered by pure energy. They cruise over sleek buildings pointed skyward and made of glass. Inside, men are working on advanced technology, and I am one of those men, one of the best and most important scientists employed there. The goal is to make everything more powerful so that we can alter all material forms, all matter on Earth, and control it, control the behavior of others, control nature. It's not for good, though. It's for dominance. We scientists are working to dominate the world."

"Interesting," I said. "You've gone into a future time." I began therapy with Hugh just as I was starting to progress my patients, and he seemed to have arrived millennia ahead without prompting.

His response surprised me: "It isn't the future at all. No. This is Atlantis."

Atlantis! The fabled realm described by dozens of writers, most famously by Edgar Cayce. It existed thirty thousand or forty thousand years ago and then disappeared. Atlantis, whose inhabitants ruled their part of the world because they alone held the secrets of all matter and all living things. Hugh had not progressed into the future; he was in a world that had vanished long before recorded history.

"My job is to change my level of consciousness and learn techniques of energy manipulation in order to transform matter," he said. He was breathing quickly and was clearly agitated by his role in this strange society.

"Transform matter by using psychic energy?" I asked, look-ing for clarification.

"Yes. Through the energy of the mind." He hesitated. "Or maybe we used crystals. Energy through crystals. I'm not sure. It's not the energy of electrical current—it's something more ad-vanced than that."

"And you're an important scientist."

"Exactly. It's what I was trained to do." He grew sad. "I want to achieve personal power. It means suppressing my spiritual side, but that's the price I must pay. Maybe I could alter my level of consciousness to an even higher vibration. That way I could advance spiritually, to approach a place beyond matter, beyond time. But I don't bother with that. My colleagues and I—what we are doing is bad. Our aim is to control the civilizations sur-rounding us, and we are succeeding. We are achieving our goal."

His life review was predictable to me. He regretted his actions and realized that he had taken the wrong path. If he had used his higher mind, his mind's energy, for good and compassionate pur-poses, not for power and self-aggrandizement, he would have led a better, happier existence. He had wasted his knowledge, wasted his power, and wasted his life.

After he had left, I wrote two notes:

"That Hugh led a previous life in Atlantis does not prove the existence of Atlantis by any means or that I believe in it. This is only his experience, and perhaps he was seeing the future after all. It might be fantasy. It might be true. The important thing is his regret that he did not use his psychic powers for higher goals. That seems to be his regret today.

"There seemed to be a higher level of technology at that time than we possess now. Perhaps many people from that time are reincarnating at the present time because our technology is, once again, advancing to the level that existed in that ancient time and we have to see if we have learned our lessons—it's the conflict be-tween the compassionate use or selfish use of our advanced powers. The last time we nearly destroyed the planet. Which option will we take now?"

At his next regression session Hugh found himself in Europe—he wasn't sure which country—in the Middle Ages. "I'm a large man with broad, powerful shoulders. I'm dressed simply in a tunic, and my hair is disheveled. I am addressing an assembly of townspeople. My eyes are piercing and wild and incredibly intense. I tell the people that they don't need to go to the church or listen to the priests to find God. 'God is in yourselves, in every one of us. You don't need those hypocrites to show you the way to Him. Everyone has access to divine wisdom. I will show you the way very simply, and you will be independent of the church and its arrogant priests. They will lose their control, which you will reclaim for yourselves.' "

Hugh was soon taken prisoner by the church authorities and was tortured to recant. But he wouldn't, no matter how cruelly he was punished. Eventually, he told me with horror, he was literally torn apart on a rack that the priests had placed in the town square, in part because of the priests' fury but also because they wanted to use him as an example to warn the townspeople not to think in dangerous ways.

In a brief review of that lifetime, he made connections back to his ancient Atlantean life, which I summarized in a later note:

"Overcompensation toward spiritual rather than selfish motives in reaction to his Atlantean life and his knowledge of the possibilities of higher levels of consciousness led Hugh to be too public and not to pay enough attention to the power of the Catholic Church at that time and its zealous elimination of heretics or anyone who attacked the Church's power, even at the lowest levels."

Hugh also made connections to his present life. "My powers were developed in Atlantis," he told me. "It's there I learned my clairvoyant, clairaudient, and telepathic skills," referring to the psychic powers of sight, hearing, and mind.

"What about the messages?" I asked.

"Those are different," he said quickly. "They come from the spirits."

"The spirits? What do you mean?"

"Spirits. Disembodied spirits. I can't be more definite." He cleared his throat. "They give me knowledge. They tell me the truth."

A familiar theme—other patients spoke of spirits—but I detected a difference. When he left, I wrote the following:

"By externalizing the origins of his knowledge to others, Hugh was magically trying to prevent an occurrence of the physical destruction visited on his body in the Middle Ages. In other words he was saying, 'This is not me. I'm just hearing it from others, even if they're spirits.' It was a kind of safety device because having psychic power is dangerous. But in a way the spirits prevented him from accessing even higher levels of his multidimensional consciousness."

Perhaps, I thought, he could access those higher levels if I progressed him to the future. He was a talented psychic. Would he perhaps be even more talented and more accurate than others if he could access what was to come? It wasn't essential to his therapy; he had learned the source of his anxiety and achieved an acceptance of his psychic powers. But still, I was curious as to what he would discover.

Would he be willing to progress to the future and take me with him? He could hardly wait.

Maybe Hugh went too deep. He seemed to be experiencing two journeys simultaneously, one into the future and the other into higher and higher levels of consciousness, to worlds and dimensions above and beyond this one.

"The next level, the one just beyond ours, isn't as dense as the one we know," he told me in a voice full of awe. "There is trouble getting there. The way is full of peril, but when we arrive, we're more mental and less physical. Everyone's telepathic. There's a higher vibration. Our bodies are lighter. Movement is easier."

In a way it was like the Atlantis he had described in his first regression. But there was more.

"I'm going up and up. At the different levels there are changes in the quality of the light. I can't describe it. It gets brighter but softer. It doesn't have color, or it has all colors. It leads to dimensions beyond light and beyond where thought could go. This level is incomprehensible to the human mind. And still I keep going. There's no end. I go beyond infinity and, if possible, even beyond that."

We both had the sense that these were positive places of great calm and beauty, though *beauty* is too humdrum a word. Hugh's description lay more in his manner than in his words. What he envisioned transcended his vocabulary, and it was the serene beauty of his face, which was no longer pinched, that served as his eloquence.

The future he described was not his personal future but the future in general. (Later, when I started progressing groups in my workshops or seminars, this was usually the case, as I'll describe in the final chapter.)

"The journey is like an airplane taking off in a thunderstorm," Hugh said. "It grows darker and darker as we reach cloud level. There's a lot of turbulence, fear, and anxiety. But then we pierce the cloud layer and come out on the other side into a brilliant sky—many shades of blue lit by an incandescent golden sun. It takes many years, many centuries to get through the clouds, which grow more ominous as the years pass. They are clouds of tragedies and calamities that will beset our civilization. But eventually, in eight hundred or a thousand years, maybe more, the clouds will disappear, the turbulence will disappear, and there will be a feeling of peacefulness, awe, and safety."

He leaned forward, confiding in me in his hypnotized state.

"The people on the other side of the storm, they have mental abilities and psychic abilities far beyond what I have now. They're telepathic." His voice was almost a whisper. "They can access all knowledge. They are mentally omnipotent."

Perhaps Hugh was describing Carl Jung's concept of the collective unconscious or what Eastern religions call the Akashic Record. In this record every action, to the tiniest detail, and every thought, no matter how trivial, of all mankind from the beginning of history is stored. Psychics may tap into this to learn the thoughts and dreams of other people, I thought. That's what he said he told the townsfolk in the medieval town. And in his future vision he had mastered what the Atlanteans were seeking. They could convert matter into energy and energy into matter, and they could transform the elemental particles into each other by harnessing the energy of consciousness. In the time of Atlantis this power was used for evil. In the Middle Ages, though Hugh did not specify it, alchemists tried to transform common minerals into gold. In the future that Hugh saw, everyone was an alchemist, and they were using their powers for good. They had come through the clouds and into the blue sky and golden light.

I think Hugh's quest is a metaphor for changing ourselves from the physical to the spiritual, and he seemed to have accomplished this in the far future. Perhaps all of us, those who are left after the "tragedies and calamities," will do the same. What he brought back from the future was this: In the time he envisioned, the physical body could change. People could come in and out of their bodies at will. They could have out-of-body experiences whenever they wished. Even death wasn't what it seemed. There was no more disease: Physical and mental illnesses had disappeared because people learned how to fix the energetic disruptions that cause disease in the physical dimensions.

I came to understand why his progressions took a dual road. In both there was a time of torment and then a paradise. Eventually, the future curved higher and higher, becoming more and more sublime until it joined the progression of higher levels of consciousness—the higher dimensions or worlds that Hugh had seen in his other journey forward. In other words, even though he was going off in two directions, he was heading for the same destination. In the first journey he went directly to higher levels of consciousness. In the second he went into future lives here on this planet. Both futures would eventually reach the highest dimensions and would meet at some point along the way. Our futures, he was saying, are like railway spurs, always leading to the main track. No matter which path we take, we are all going to the same place, and that place is a joy beyond all words and all human comprehension.

In his present life Hugh no longer feels different because he knows that his talents are possessed by all of us, although they are latent in most. He feels better about himself and privileged that he has been allowed glimpses into higher worlds. His work is much clearer to him, and he seems to receive information from higher levels now. He no longer attributes his knowledge to "discrete and external spirits" because of the fear carried over from the Middle Ages. He knows his powers lie within himself. He is happier, and that is the best measure of his progress. The clarity of his psychic readings reflects a clarity in his intention to help others, in his will to transform despair into hope, and in his life. He has become the alchemist he set out to be millennia ago.

I've included his story in my discussion of compassion not because he needed to learn it on his road to immortality, but because he had a superabundance of it. He felt sorrow and love for all who approached him, and in so doing he gave up too much of himself. Without compassion no one can ascend to high planes in the lives to come, but like all the virtues discussed in this book, it is part of a whole. One must learn compassion for others but also for oneself.

* * *

Chitra, thirty-five, also gave compassion without reward. A molecular research biologist, she spent her days in the lab and her evenings with her sickly and demanding mother with whom she had lived for ten years. There was no time for a social life or, indeed, for a life of any kind of her own.

She was the youngest child in an Indian family that had come to America when she was young, and given the Hindu tradition in which she was raised, she was expected to be the caregiver for her mother. A brother and his wife could not be expected to do this, nor could her married older sister who had two children of her own. Chitra had been married to a much older man—an arranged marriage—but her husband had died, leaving her with no children. As a result, the care of her mother fell to her.

When she came to me, she complained that her mother's dependency and overprotectiveness was suffocating her; in fact, her breathing was labored, and she had trouble getting out her words. Hindi was her first language, but she spoke fluent English, as did her mother. She dressed only in saris except at work when she wore jeans and sweaters under her lab coat. She was a curious and delightful mixture of two cultures, though I doubt she was amused. It was the older culture that kept her from enjoying the younger.

Many Hindus believe in reincarnation, but for them it is an intellectual belief, part of their religion. Its use as a therapeutic tool is virtually unknown. Chitra may or may not have believed in past lives; she was reticent when I broached the subject. But she readily agreed to a regression. After two weeks of practicing relaxation and hypnotic techniques, she was able to enter a moderate trance state. Her impressions were hazy and her words halting.

"I'm in India . . . a prostitute but not really a prostitute. . . . I travel with the army which is fighting my enemies. . . . I don't know what year it is. . . . Not so long ago . . . I am told that I am needed by the soldiers. . . . They are all-important. . . . It is my army, my people. . . . They have to be cared for. . . . I feed them

. . . satisfy their sexual needs. . . . I *hate* what I have to do. . . . I can see myself dying. . . . I am still very young. . . . Yes, I am dying . . . dying giving birth to a child."

That was all. In her life review she realized she didn't want to linger in such a place. Helping the soldiers fight India's enemies was not a higher good at all. It was a convention devised by selfish and cruel men, and as a woman she was trapped, doomed.

The second regression was just as brief. "I am a woman . . . sacrificial robes. . . . I must be killed to ensure a good harvest. . . . Maybe my death will protect my people from enemies . . . from natural disasters. . . . I am told it is a great honor to die. . . . I and my family will be rewarded in the afterlife. . . . There is a sword over my head. . . . It strikes."

In both cases she had trouble breathing, and each time I brought her quickly back to the present. Chitra needed to learn from these lifetimes, but not in great detail. She went straight to the traumas, and when we talked about them, she realized that violence is antithetical to spiritual concepts. Promises of later rewards were self-serving lies by the generals or religious elders whose power was based on ignorance, deception, and fear.

We discovered the link in the two lives and their relevance to Chitra's present situation: In both regressions she had been forced to sacrifice her own life, her own goals, her own happiness for some "higher" good. And, in effect, the sacrifice killed her, as it was killing her now.

Chitra's mother had a past life memory as well, though she never came into my office. Excited about the work we were doing, Chitra brought home my regression CDs and was practicing at home, just as I encourage all my patients to do. Her mother, listening, saw herself as a young Indian wife three centuries ago. In that life Chitra was her mother's deeply beloved husband, the focus of her existence. But soon the man died, probably from the venom of a snakebite. When Chitra's mother came back to the present, she understood that she had clung to Chitra, her daughter, and explained it to Chitra as a reaction to her loss centuries ago. Her mother's dependency and overprotectiveness, Chitra now realized, had their roots not in this lifetime but in a different one, and she was able to be more forgiving.

Her mother began to change. Slowly, for she was overcoming years of habit, she became less clinging, less protective. She became more open to spending time with her other children, and she was even willing to let Chitra start a social life, despite the possibility that it would lead Chitra into a relationship that would interfere with her dependency. This in turn led to an improvement in Chitra's outlook. For the first time she could look forward without dread, and she let me lead her into the future.

Chitra experienced what I took to be three future lives during a single progression. In the first she saw herself as the mother and principal caregiver of a young child with severe muscular, skeletal, and neurological deficits. The family dynamic required Chitra to expend most of her time and energy on the little girl with little return. Her husband in that life had withdrawn emotionally and often physically; he simply couldn't deal with the tragedy. Thus the flow of compassion, love, and energy seemed to me unidirectionally outward, with Chitra giving but never receiving.

In a second future life Chitra suffered severe physical injuries in a vehicle accident. "You couldn't really call it a car," she told me. "It was more like a giant flying cylinder with windows. Anyway, its programming malfunctioned, and *wham!*—it crashed head-on into a tree." Chitra was paralyzed and had to receive extensive physical and psychological rehabilitation. "The technical levels of medicine are advanced," she said with some satisfaction, "but regeneration of my nervous system tissue, both brain and spinal cord, took more than a year." Chitra smiled. "The hospital staff was superb, but recovery was very difficult. I'm not sure I would have made it without the love of my family—I have an adoring husband and two boys and a girl—and of my friends. And the flowers! People called my hospital room the Garden of Allah."

Here, I thought, was the reverse of the first life. Again, compassion, love, and energy were unidirectional, but this time they were flowing in.

In her third future, Chitra was a surgeon, specializing in orthopedics and neurology. "I work with rods or crystals," she explained when I pointed out how uncommon it was to have two such different areas of expertise. "They emit a light, an energy, that has a remarkable healing effect, whether it be bones or brain. They also cause a sound energy that helps in the regeneration of muscles, limbs, and ligaments."

Chitra derived huge satisfaction from the results of her knowledge and skills. There was also positive feedback not only from her patients and their families but from her professional colleagues. Her family life, too, was happy and flourishing. In this life she seemed to have achieved the proper balance of inflow and outflow. She was able to love others as well as herself.

Chitra told me that she reviewed this third life from a higher perspective, meaning that she had risen to a new level. She was still in a hypnotized state when she said this, but then she suddenly stopped. "I don't know how this life is going to end. It's puzzling. I'll just have to leave it. Now!" As always, she was not one to linger in past or future lives.

Suddenly she was back in the present, animated and stimulated by her voyages. "All the lives, past and present, are connected," she explained, "as is this life and the past life my mother described. What I've got to do is balance compassion, balance love, which must be received as well as given." Her determination was palpable. "My life's goals will never be sacrificed again—not because of cultural values, individual circumstances, or guilt," she said. She was able to express her anger and resentment toward her mother and her siblings for trapping her in the caregiver role—despite the cultural taboos prohibiting such rebellion—and by so doing freed herself.

We went back to the third of her future lives, and this time she was able to see its end: death at an old age of natural causes. In her life review the significance that eluded me became clear to her. "The three future lives weren't sequential or linear," she explained. "They're manifestations of probable futures based on what I do in this life."

In a sense they were parallel futures that flowed simultaneously; the one she ended up in would stem from the content of the remainder of her life now. In fact, there were "a multitude of possible futures," she told me, "all variations of the three I witnessed. And it's not only my consciousness but the collective thoughts and actions of the entire human population that will have a role in shaping the one that turns out to be the actual one. If we consciously embrace compassion, empathy, love, patience, and forgiveness, the future world will be incredibly different than if we don't."

Her language had changed markedly. She no longer spoke in short, choppy sentences. Her more sophisticated words and ideas reflected a connection to a higher level of consciousness. This wise young woman had much to teach me.

"We have much more power to positively influence our individual future lives as well as the remaining future of our present life than we do to influence the planetary or collective future," I noted after she left. "But our individual futures express themselves in the collective future, and the actions of everyone will determine which of a myriad possible futures we will come back to. If Chitra continued stuck in her present family pattern, then she might have to experience a future as the paralysis victim forced to receive love. If she just gave up, abruptly ending her relationship with her mother, abandoning her without a reasonable compromise, she might have had to come back as the mother of the seriously impaired child. Because that is how it works: We face similar situations again and again as we seek to learn the proper balance between giving and receiving, between sacrifice and compassion for ourselves—until we achieve the state of harmony. Given what she had learned and having recognized that balance, Chitra would come back as the orthopedic/neurological surgeon, but she could be born into a world of more or less violence, more or less compassion and loving, depending on the harmony others attain. If enough of us can somehow elevate the consciousness of humankind—if we can commit to changing the collective future by improving our individual futures—we can actually change the future of the entire world and all its inhabitants."

Compassion is, as I've said, related to empathy. It is also related to love, in that it comes from the heart, just as love does. Three simple exercises will help you reach that place in your heart where compassion, empathy, and love coexist, as will the psychometry exercise I provided in chapter 3.

A Tear of Joy

Relax, using the same method described in chapter 3. When you are in a relaxed state, remember a time in your life when a tear of joy came to your eye. (You might remember several times.) I'm not talking about when you won the lottery or your team won the World Series; I mean a time associated with something loving in your life. It can be a moment when someone unexpectedly did a good deed for you, such as volunteering to take care of your children so you and your spouse could have a private weekend together, or visiting you when you were sick. Or it can be a time when you did a good deed for somebody else, an action coming not from a sense of responsibility but from the heart. The point is that the giver—you or a friend or stranger—acted out of compassion, with no expectation of reward. The more you do this exercise, the more the compassionate moments will be linked, one to the next, and the more easily a tear or tears will come. By bringing compassionate memories freshly into your consciousness you will increase your capacity for joy, happiness, and further acts of compassion.

Interconnectedness

In a relaxed state, look into someone's eyes. If you see that person looking back at you, that is the everyday event, so go deeper. Look beyond what lies at the surface of his or her eyes. Try to see the *soul* looking back at you, and if you find it, you'll see there is more depth in that person than just a physical body. You'll know that all people have a soul just as you do and that their soul and your soul are connected. If you see your own soul looking back, you'll have reached a deeper level because you'll see that we're all of one substance and of one soul. How is it possible not to feel compassion then, for in treating another humanely, are you not treating yourself? By loving another, are you not loving yourself?

The Humanity of Others

A variation of the above is to visualize the humanity of other people—friends, family, or strangers. They are not just a name or a trait ("My aunt Maude never stops talking!" "That homeless person is filthy!") but are multidimensional, made up of a complex of factors, just as you are. They have mothers, fathers, children, and loved ones. It doesn't matter what their nationality is or whether they claim to be your foe. They experience joy, love, fear, anxieties, despair, and sorrow exactly as you and I do. They were children once, laughing and playing with their balls, their dolls, their pets, their games, when they were trusting. I have my patients visualize as children their enemies or people they hate or are angry at. That's just a start. See them as young lovers, as parents, as people who have won and lost, who have experienced birth and death, victory and tragedy. Really see the details. Particularize. By so doing you are not seeing them as a group but as individuals who have experienced everything that you have experienced. It is easy to hate groups because they don't have individual qualities. If you follow this exercise, you'll give up hate because it is harder to hate fully rounded individuals and impossible to hate souls. I had compassion for that Russian soldier, the man I was supposed to fear. He had a soul, I realized. His soul was mine.

Compassion and empathy aren't learned overnight; life's lessons are not simple. Another factor must come into play as we ascend toward immortality: patience.

CHAPTER 6

Paul: Patience and Understanding

T HE BUDDHISTS HAVE AN EXPRESSION: "Don't push the river. It will travel at its own speed anyway."

For purposes of spiritual evolution, it helps to envision time as a river, though we should measure it not chronologically, as we do now, but in lessons learned on our road to immortality. So don't push the river of time. You're just going to splash around impotently; that is, you can thrash against the current or flow with it peacefully. Impatience robs us of joy, peace, and happiness. We want what we want, and we want it now. Nowhere is this more evident than in twenty-first-century America. But that's not how the universe is engineered. Things come to us when we are ready. Before we are born, we look over the landscape of the life to come, only to forget it after birth. We hurry in the present, worrying only about fixing the now, but as adults in our present lives we should recognize there is a right and a wrong time. For example, why did Catherine turn up in my life that year and not two years earlier or later? And why, when I asked her about the future, did she say, "Not now"?

After *Only Love Is Real,* my book about soul mates, came out, I received a letter from a woman that read, "Well, I met my soul mate, but now I'm married. I have three children. *He's* married and has two children. Why didn't we meet when we were teenagers?"

Because destiny had a different plan. They were *supposed* to meet later. People come into our lives at certain times for various reasons having to do with lessons to be learned. It is not a coincidence that they didn't meet at a much earlier age when they did not have other commitments. I think the reason people meet later is to learn about love in many different ways and about how to balance this with responsibility and commitment. They'll meet again in a different lifetime. They must be patient.

One woman patient committed suicide in an earlier life because her husband, a sergeant in World War I, was listed as missing in action and she was sure he was dead. In fact, he had been taken prisoner and returned to America after the war, only to discover the fate of his wife. In her life or the ones following, this woman will learn patience if she remembers the lesson of the past one.

Friends of mine, high school sweethearts, went separate ways into unhappy marriages. When they met again forty years later, they had an affair, divorced their present spouses, and married. It was as though no time had elapsed. The same feelings were there, with the same intensity. I did regressions with both of them, and they were together in past lives as well. This coming together of people late in life who had been together in past lives happens a lot.

Psychological patience rather than physical patience is the key. Time as we measure it can go fast or slowly. Tom Brady, the quarterback for the New England Patriots football team, thinks a minute is more than enough time in which to engineer the winning score. When I am stuck in a traffic jam, it seems like an eternity. But if we internalize time as the endless river it is, then impatience disappears. "I don't want to die yet," a patient tells me. "There are many more things I need to do." Yes, but he'll have infinite time in which to do them.

Patience is related to understanding because the more you understand a person or a situation or an experience—or yourself—the less likely it is that you'll have a knee-jerk reaction and do something hurtful to yourself or others. Let's say your spouse comes home and yells at you for some minor infraction—perhaps you forgot to walk the dog or buy the milk. The impatient response is to yell back. But *be patient! Understand!* Maybe the anger coming at you has nothing to do with you but is the result of a bad day at the office, an oncoming cold, a migraine, an allergy, or even a bad mood. As the spouse you are the safe person; he or she can vent at you knowing that nothing serious will happen even if you flare up in return. But if you are patient, you might get at the cause of the anger and then dissipate it. If your response is a patient one and you understand that there is a hidden reason behind the explosion, then it is no great trick restoring harmony.

You'll need the ability to detach, to see from a distance, to achieve a higher perspective to do so. As you'll learn in chapter 11, meditation and contemplation are the handmaidens of patience, for they help you achieve distance. As you develop the ability to be quiet, to be introspective, and to listen, patience invariably develops. If nations were more patient, there would be fewer wars because there would be more time for diplomacy, for dialogue, and, again, for understanding. Nations rarely strive for patience, but people should. If you train yourself to be patient, you will recognize its importance when it arrives and make progress on the spiritual path toward immortality.

Sometimes, however, you may have to wait until you see the future to fully recognize its power.

Paul had money, no doubt about that. He had made a fortune in copper gutters for seaside residences, and he had also invested wisely. But as he told me in our first session, his money was doing him no good, and he felt like a failure. His twenty-two-year-old daughter, Alison, had leukemia, and her chances of recovery were, as he put it, "slim to none." His money could pay for the best doctors, the best drugs, and the best advice—but not for miracles. He was frequently depressed and saw his life as useless despite his monetary success.

Usually I can take a patient's history in one session or less. With Paul it took two, not only because the history was complicated but because he was so reluctant to give it. He was fifty, tall, fit, silver-haired, and silver-tongued. His blue eyes looked at me with the openness that one sees in people with nothing to hide or in con men. In Paul's case I suspected the latter. (It turned out he was conning himself, not me.) His smile was broad, his teeth white in a perfectly tanned face, and his nails professionally manicured. He wore a white Ralph Lauren sport shirt, tan slacks with a knife-edge crease, and enviable leather sandals.

"I'm not sure I should be here," he said as we shook hands and I got my first hit of those eyes.

"Many people feel that way. Psychiatry can seem forbidding. Who wants to reveal his soul to a stranger? Besides, people think, incorrectly, that there's a touch of the occult in what I do."

"Occult. Exactly. And—forgive me if I'm rude—this business of taking people into their past lives . . ."

"Weird," I agreed, smiling. "It took me years to believe that some patients weren't somehow making up their stories despite all evidence to the contrary. But I assure you that I have no occult powers and that even if some of my patients were fantasizing, they still got better."

He seemed to accept this, for he nodded and sat down across from me and talked about Alison.

"I'm afraid my wife, my other daughter, and my son—all three of them together—are sabotaging her treatment," he said, more distraught than angry.

"In what way?"

"Alison is a vegetarian, but she needs meat to keep her strong. Instead, my family encourages her to take megavitamins and minerals and—Jesus!—tomatoes and wheat germ. She's into yoga and meditation, too. I suppose that's all right—can't hurt her—but they want me to join the party."

"They're simply taking a holistic approach," I said mildly.

"Well, I want them to join mine."

"Which is?"

"Aggressive medicine. Radiation. Chemo. The works."

"Isn't she getting these?"

"Sure she is. My insistence. I'm calling the shots. But to waste her time with that other nonsense—to think it's going to cure her—is insane. I asked her to stop it, but she won't." He lowered his head to his hands and massaged his eyes. "She's disobeyed me from the time she was a toddler."

"What about your other kids? Were they disobedient, too?"

"Nah. Good as gold. Always were. My wife, too. Always will be."

I was developing quite an admiration for Alison. Her "disobedience" sounds like spunk, I thought. She's probably the only one in the family who has stood up to him. Maybe he is so upset because the others are taking her side for once.

"There is a great debate about holistic medicine," I told him. "Great societies, such as the Chinese, put their faith in it. They believe—"

"In acupuncture!" he practically shouted. "She's trying that, too. And the kids—yes, and my wife, too—are letting it happen."

I believe that some forms of holistic medicine are effective, particularly when used in conjunction with orthodox medical treatment. I said, "As long as she is getting the proper medical treatment, why be uptight about it? Hope, you know, is a factor in recovery. If she thinks the acupuncture is helping, maybe that is value enough."

"I suppose so," he grumbled. He left, obviously unsatisfied.

I wondered if he would return, but he was back for his appointment three days later, this time with a new complaint: her boyfriend.

"And you object?"

"I certainly do!"

"Why?"

"He isn't good enough for her. None of them are. He won't stay for the long haul."

I was beginning to see a pattern. "What does she think of you?"

"She loves me, I suppose."

"Only suppose?"

He thought for a while before answering. "It's funny. I feel awkward around her. Can't tease her the way I can the other kids. When I go to hug her—or maybe it's the other way around—I seem to freeze."

"Yet you love her."

"My God, yes!"

"Have you told her?"

He bowed his head. "I don't seem to be able to find a way. We're always squabbling. She says I pick on her, but all I'm trying to do is make sure she's safe."

Keeping her under control seemed to me a poor way of showing love. "What about her other boyfriends?" I asked.

"Hopeless."

"How so?"

"Not smart enough. Oafs, really. All testosterone and souped-up cars. Or nerds—too smart, no balls. Actually, Phil is the best of them. He did show up at the hospital the last time she had to stay over. None of the others would do that. The last time he visited, I told him not to come back."

"Was that the first time you said it?"

"To his face. But I've told Alison she couldn't see him again."

I smiled. "But she was 'disobedient.' "

He shrugged. The answer was obvious.

"Don't you think it would give her pleasure to go on seeing him? After all, if she doesn't get better—"

He interrupted with a roar. "Stop right there! Goddamn it, I'll make sure she gets better even if I have to die in her place."

After the two sessions of history taking and discussion, I was eager to look deeper at Paul's relationship with Alison. Something accounted for his overly protective behavior, both toward her and toward himself. Perhaps the answer lay in a past life. He resisted at first, but finally, with his family's blessing and encouragement, and because Alison was so ill, he agreed. It took longer than usual to hypnotize him because of his active left brain and his need to stay in control, but eventually he reached a deep level.

"It's 1918," he told me. "I'm in a northern city, New York or Boston. I'm twenty-three years old. I'm a very proper young man, following my father's career as a banker, and I'm in love, wildly in love, with the wrong girl. She's a singer and dancer, a real stunner. I've talked to her occasionally after the show, but I've never revealed my feelings. I know she's—" He paused, a look of incredulity spreading over his face. "It's my daughter Alison!"

He sat silently for a moment, remembering. Then he said: "I've talked to her, told her I love her, and—blessed day—she loves me, too. Can you believe it? She loves me, too! I know my parents won't approve, but it doesn't matter. I'll defy them. She's everything to me."

Once more his expression changed. He grew sad. "She died," he whispered. "Died in the epidemic, and with her death, our dreams died, too, and I've lost all joy, all hope, all pleasure. There will never be another love like ours."

I asked him to go slightly forward in that life. He saw himself as a dour, angry man, old at forty when, blind drunk, he drove his car off the road and died.

I brought him back, and we discussed the connection the past life had to the present. Two patterns emerged. One involved magical thinking: In this life, if he didn't tell Alison he loved her, she would be safe; she wouldn't die as she had in 1918. The second

SAME SOUL, MANY BODIES ———— 101

was a counterphobic mechanism, the same impulse that makes someone quit if he thinks he's about to be fired. In Paul's case it meant that if he kept an emotional distance from Alison, he would be protected from pain, grief, and despair if he should lose her. So he backed away from her, picked fights, criticized constantly, and interfered with her boyfriends. Her current illness made him relive the panic he had felt nearly a century earlier. He knew, he said as he left my office, that as part of her treatment he would have to confront his fears and avow his love. Some part of him understood that the body-mind connection, well known to immunologists, had been validated.

Paul's fears were already eased slightly because he had lost Alison before and had suffered for it. Both had died, yet both had come back to this life. He was still distraught at the probability of her death, but he allowed himself now to feel his love for her. He didn't need to protect himself so severely, to the detriment of both of them.

His first response to his impulse of unconditional love was to call Phil and tell him he was free to visit Alison in the hospital or at home as much as he wanted. Alison was thrilled, and Phil could hardly believe Paul's change in attitude. As the young lovers' relationship deepened, Paul became more and more welcoming. He realized that Alison's happiness was more important than his protection of her.

Something wondrous was happening. As Phil's and Alison's love grew, and as Paul was able to express his love by his actions, Alison's immune system went into high gear. Love became a vital medicine in her fight against cancer.

One week later Paul returned for his second regression. This time he was a nineteenth-century woman, the wife of a fisherman, living on the coast of New England. Once again anxiety and dread filled his life.

"He's not coming back this time."

"Who's not coming back?"

"My husband. He goes on these trips—sometimes they last for months—and I'm sure he won't return."

"He has taken these trips before?"

"Yes."

"And come back before?"

"Yes."

"Then why not this time?"

"Because this time he's dead. I can feel it." He took in great gulps of air. "My women friends try to cheer me—they have fisherman husbands, too—but they can't. I'm going mad with worry."

His fear was so palpable that I asked if he wanted to be brought back to the present. He held up his hand. "Wait. There's news." He began to wail. "The boat capsized. All aboard were lost. I was right. He's dead. My darling is dead. There is no life for me now."

The grieving New England woman quickly sank into a depression. She stopped eating, couldn't sleep, and soon died of heartbreak. Her soul left her body, but it stayed watching for a long time. The woman had died the week before her husband returned to the town. He had been rescued with two of his mates, and they had spent their time slowly recuperating in the home of a farmer's widow until they were strong enough to make their way back.

The woman's (Paul's) husband in that life was Alison.

In the New England wife's life review, a new theme emerged: patience. She saw that if she had waited, not despaired—in effect, not killed herself—she would have been reunited with her husband and been happy. When I brought Paul back, he saw that patience was a missing element in his other lives as well. The Paul who had died in an automobile crash had actually found his love

again—here, in this life, in his daughter. Knowledge of subsequent lives might have stopped him from drinking, the cause of
the crash, and he might have had a fulfilled life then while waiting
for the return of his beloved. In this life he realized that if he had
not inserted himself into Alison's life the way he did, if he had let
her be and allowed her to love freely, then her cancer might not
have been as overwhelming. She might have had more energy and
more will to fight it. Even now, he thought, it might not be too
late.

The following week's session began with a progress report.
Alison was feeling better. Her doctors were encouraged. All the
different approaches—the standard treatment, the holistic approach, Phil's presence, and Paul's changed behavior—seemed to
be working. Paul told me he had hugged Alison the night before,
fully and wholeheartedly, and told her that he loved her. She had
responded by hugging him back, saying she loved him, too, and
bursting into tears. "What's more," he said, smiling, "I even
hugged Phil. But I didn't tell him I loved him." It was a huge moment for him, and he attributed it to the regressions. He asked me
to lead him back again.

Several centuries ago in the ancient culture of India, Paul had
a lifetime as a lower caste girl. Alison was Paul's close friend in
that life. Though they were not related, she was "as close or
closer than any sister." The two were dependent on each other for
emotional survival; they shared their thoughts and wishes, joy
and pain. Since they were at the bottom of the social ladder, their
lives were very hard, but they managed by helping each other
every day.

Then, Paul told me bitterly, Alison fell in love. The young
man, whom Paul recognized as his own wife (Alison's mother) in
this life, was of a higher caste; nevertheless, they had an affair.
Paul warned Alison of the dreadful consequences if they were
caught together. Alison said her "sister" was just jealous and
went around her village boasting of the young man's love for her.

The boy's family found out, and Alison was murdered by his father for disgracing their caste. The loss devastated Paul; he remained bitter, grieving, and angry for the rest of his/her short life.

As he floated above his body in that past life, Paul could connect that life to his current one and to the lives he remembered from his first two regressions. The recurrent pattern of the traumatic loss of love through death had led to his current fears and protective mechanisms. He had also learned the value of patience. In his Indian life, too, he had shunned pleasure and joy when they might have been his if he had known that Alison would return not once but many times. There were other lessons as well: the danger of rushing to judgment, the folly of experiencing events without perspective, and the sometimes mortal risks of losing control. He was learning to let go of his fears of death and loss. More positively, he grasped the concept of the supreme value of love and its healing effects. Love is an absolute, he understood, and cannot be diminished by time or distance. It can be obscured by fear, but its brilliance is never really lessened. Fear closes the mind, love opens the heart and dissolves fear.

I wondered aloud whether to progress Paul into the future, but we held back for a long time. He and I were both reluctant to look ahead in his current life—he because he couldn't bear the thought of finding out that Alison's cancer would eventually defeat her, and I because I was concerned that his anxiety over Alison's illness would distort his future memories. At last we decided that looking into a future life, as opposed to seeing ahead in this one, held no such risks. So in our last session together, that's where we went—to a future life.

It was an unusual progression because Paul saw not a continuous narrative but a series of three snapshots, like pictures in a slide show. The glimpses were vivid, however, and filled with strong

emotion. He saw himself older in this lifetime, successful and fulfilled thanks to the fact that his daughter had been cured. He saw
Alison alive and well at age sixty-seven in the future of her current lifetime. He also saw himself reincarnating as Alison's
grandson, being received with love and joy into Alison's future
family. (When I asked him how far in the future this snapshot
was, he said, "Forty-five years." I was concerned that this meant
Paul's death was imminent in his present life, but he had no problems with the math. I was forgetting that in this instance time is
past, present, and future in one.) Afterward we discussed his progression.

"Don't the episodes seem to you like wish fulfillment?" I
asked.

"Not at all. They could be. Now that you bring it up, I can see
why you'd think so, but what I saw wasn't how my imagination
works. I've never had visions like these before. They seem very
real."

That he saw himself as Alison's grandson gave credence to his
beliefs, though in my mind the memories were a little too "perfect." Even the Alison-grandson relationship could be explained
by his intense desire to win her love in the present. Nevertheless,
he believed the scenes were real, and that was all that mattered.

"My next life wouldn't have been possible if Alison hadn't
been healed," he said.

The statement brought me up short. Alison was still very
sick—remissions such as hers can be devastatingly fleeting—and
I wondered what would happen to Paul if she died. Perhaps he
had truly learned patience, I reflected. Perhaps it would be
enough that he knew he would meet her again in a future life.
There was no reason to shake his equilibrium. He was a different
man from the self-hating smoothie who had first walked into my
office. Besides, maybe what he saw was true.

"She might not have gotten better without you," I told him.

He was startled. "How do you mean?"

"For one thing, you chose to allow Alison's boyfriend to visit and left her free to fall in love. For another, you gave up your control and allowed yourself to love her openly and fully. Among other benefits, including the benefit to you, her immune system's response to that dual love may have been instrumental in fighting her cancer. I believe it was."

"Along with the medicine," he said.

"Along with the medicine. But the medicine hadn't worked before you changed."

"And I changed thanks to you."

It felt strange to hear him speak so humbly. "I just pointed the way. The important thing to realize is that you exercised the most important of all human attributes: You used your free will."

Paul could have chosen to remain stubborn and inflexible. He could also have chosen to decline the past life therapy and then not have gained the understanding and insights he obtained. If he had been closed-minded, dictatorial, or impatient, Alison might not have gone into remission. He had instead chosen the path of courage, the path of love.

Over the following months, with Phil and Paul joining the rest of her family at her side, Alison's improvement led to a remission. Her cancer seemed to be gone, just as Paul had seen in his future life. That life had reassured him in the present. Maybe his optimism and his certainty, along with his love, helped her get well.

Paul's story demonstrates the essential role that patience plays in our passage toward immortality. Inner peace is impossible without patience. Wisdom requires patience. Spiritual growth implies the mastery of patience. Patience allows the unfolding of destiny to proceed at its own unhurried pace.

When we are impatient, we create misery for ourselves and for others. We rush to rash judgments and act without considering the consequences of what we do. Our choices are forced and often incorrect, and we are liable to pay a steep price.

Paul could have avoided heartache and premature death in his past lives if he had been more patient. It took him until this century, this time, to understand that his present life and all those to come would be more harmonious and more fulfilled if he did not try to push the river of time.

CHAPTER 7

Emily, Joyce, Roberta, and Anne: Nonviolence

A THIRTY-YEAR-OLD WOMAN NAMED EMILY, living in a previous life as part of a nomadic tribe in Central America, was
killed in a mud slide in that earlier life, the result of an earthquake in 1634. Her frantic husband tried desperately to save her,
but his efforts were futile. For her it was the end of a life of hard-
ship. The tribe spent most of its time searching for water, and
Emily, when I regressed her to the time before her death, remembered unending physical labor. The violence of nature was a
given in her life. She spent her days in constant fear not only for
her own safety but for the safety of the seventy others in her tribe.

In this current life Emily had a terror of being caught in an
earthquake, trapped in an elevator, or imprisoned. At a workshop she told me that her husband, her daughter (who was her
sister in the earlier life—again, those who are vital to us often appear in our past lives), and her present-day sister had been mem-
bers of the ancient tribe, and once again she feared for them as
for herself. The events of 9/11 traumatized her—no more severe
"earthquake" could be imagined. She became very, very ill, barely
able to leave her home.

Another woman at that workshop named Joyce, listening to

her story, began to sob, and I asked her why she was so moved. She had detailed, vivid dreams of 9/11, she said, only they occurred on the night of September 10. Since coming to the workshop she had been drawn to Emily. She had never met her but, without knowing why, had followed her for two days without speaking to her. Now she knew why, and she also knew why she, like Emily, had been afraid to leave her house. She was a successful woman with a worldwide public relations network, but since 9/11 she had not been able to go to her branch offices outside New York, and her business was suffering. The two women embraced, finding solace in each other.

In Emily's case it was the violence of nature that caused a trauma which persisted over many centuries. In Joyce's the violence was man-made and might remain with her in future lives unless psychotherapy eased her fear. Their stories stayed with me, for I abhor violence: To me it is one of the most terrible plagues of our planet. If violence is natural—a hurricane or an earthquake—we must accept it and understand that it probably happens for a reason. But violence caused by our own hands and wills, whether toward other humans or against the planet itself, places us individually and collectively in jeopardy. Anger management is a start toward preventing it. As we saw in chapter 2, without his regressions, George might easily have injured one of his colleagues or a family member since some of violence's worst effects can be visited on the violent person's family, friends, and colleagues. I have dozens of similar cases of people who were violent or suffered violence in past lives and had to experience the effects on themselves and on others in later lives, including this one.

Roberta came to see me at the urging of her husband, Tom, a thirty-eight-year-old accountant who developed a successful practice working freelance for small businesses. I had met him at a fund-raiser for Mount Sinai Medical Center. Roberta, six years younger, was also successful, a vice president in the public relations department of a major airline. She came in early one bright winter morning, Tom at her side.

Her blond curly hair, sparkling in the office light, surrounded an oval face and gave her a Little Orphan Annie look, the impression of youth offset by piercing wise blue eyes and a wide, sensuous mouth delicately lipsticked in light red. She was slim, and her hand was soft when it shook mine.

Tom had told me that they were having trouble conceiving, and I presumed the psychological ramifications of that were what had brought them to me. I was wrong.

"Tom is going to leave me," she blurted as soon as he had left the room and I had finished taking down the details of age, address, profession, and family. But when we met at the fund-raiser, Tom said that Roberta was his "reason for being," hardly the remark of a man about to ditch his wife.

"What makes you think so?" I asked. "Has he said anything? Intimated in any way that he's—"

"Oh, no," she said quickly. "Nothing like that." She paused, gnawed at a nail, and looked at me shyly. "I just know it."

"There's no objective event? It's an internal feeling?"

She shrugged. "You'd probably call it a fantasy, but it's so real, it haunts me. I can't sleep. It's all I think about."

"And when you talk to Tom about it?"

"He tells me I'm being silly. I stopped asking Tom because he'd think I was still silly or even paranoid, and that would prompt him to leave me quicker."

This kind of circular thinking is common in patients who have lost some grounding with reality. "Then how do you act toward him?"

Her eyes looked toward the floor. "Mostly I cling to him even though I don't think he likes it. That makes me mad, so I push him away. He and I both hate it that I'm so dependent. He says I should trust him, have confidence in him, in us. I know I should, but I can't."

"What does Tom say when you tell him you can't?"

"Nothing. His silence is the worst." I could see her tremble, though her voice remained strong. Obviously, she was feeling deep emotion. "He's a good man. When I'm happy, he's happy, but when I'm sad, he gets sad too."

"And when you're angry and push him away?"

"I think he gets angry too, but he doesn't like to show it. Mostly he tries to get me out of my moods—jolly me out of them like I'm some kind of invalid or emotional cripple."

"He tells me you're having trouble conceiving," I said.

Her expression grew sad. "Yes."

"You've seen a doctor?"

"Of course. He could find nothing wrong with either of us."

"What about in vitro fertilization?"

This was a safe topic. Her voice grew steadier. "It's an option, but we don't want to do it unless the doctor feels it's our only choice. I'm sensitive to hormones of all kinds. Put me next to a bee, and I'm in terror of anaphylactic shock."

"What about adoption?"

"Again, an option, a last resort. I want *his* child."

"And he wants yours?"

"Absolutely."

"Your sex life is healthy?"

She blushed. "Robust."

"Good." We were silent for a while. I must have been smiling because those penetrating eyes caught mine, and she was suddenly angry.

"What's so funny?"

"You're both trying to have a baby. Your sex life is . . . robust. He's given no hint that he wants to leave you. I know for a fact that Tom says you're his reason for being. Why not take him at his word?"

"Because of the fear," she said gravely.

"Fear of what?"

"Of being abandoned." She began to cry. "I can't think of anything worse."

* * *

Here was a classic argument for regression therapy. There was nothing in Roberta's life that pointed to abandonment by someone she loved, but her terror was so great that it seemed clear she had been abandoned at some previous time. She loved Tom dearly, and he knew it. Her behavior and fears made no sense in the context of what I knew about their relationship. Maybe, I told her, we could find the source of her fears in another time, another life.

"Oh," she said. "If we could, how marvelous!"

She was soon under, and it did not take long for us to find a link.

"It's 849," she said with enormous sorrow, "the year I died. I live in a nice house, one of the best in our village. I have a husband I love very much—he is my life—and I'm four months pregnant with our first child. It's a difficult pregnancy. I'm often sick, and it's hard for me to work. I'm only comfortable when I'm lying down."

A look of anguish crossed her face, and she raised her hands protectively over her eyes. "We're in imminent danger of attack. There's an invading army at our gates. All the townspeople, men and women, are armed against them, prepared to fight for the town." Tears came. "I'm too weak to fight. My husband says I'm to stay home and that if he sees the battle is going badly, he'll come back for me and take me south to the village of his ancestors. I beg him to take me now, but he says he must fight. It's his duty."

"How do you feel about that?" I asked.

"Sad. Very sad. Who'll look after me?"

Her anguish was evident. "Do you want to stop the regression?"

"No. To go on."

Deeply hypnotized, she began to breathe heavily, and her body tensed in her chair.

"He's gone," she told me. "I can hear the shouts and screams of the battle. I pace the floor, waiting. I'm frightened, worried about my unborn baby. The door bursts open. 'Thank God,' I say, only it isn't my husband, it's the invaders. They rape me. An invader slashes at me with a sword. Slashes again. The sword strikes my womb. The baby dies. I fall. There's blood everywhere. Another slash, this at my throat." She gave a strangled cry. "I'm dead."

When I brought her back, she looked at me with horror. "My husband," she said. "He was Tom. My Tom. My love. He left me there to die."

It was as though sunshine had left the room.

As we've seen in other cases, present-life relatives of the patient appear in past lives, but their relationship to the patient is often changed. A daughter can become a grandmother, a father a sister, a brother, or a child. We learn from our relationships. People came back together again and again to resolve issues and to learn about love in all forms.

Sometimes, as in Roberta's case, the relationships are the same. Her husband, Tom, in this life was her husband in the ninth century as well, and he abandoned her—or did he? I wondered if it would be possible to regress Tom into the same time and place to find out what had happened to him that day. Why had he abandoned her? What was his life like after the death of his wife and unborn child? In the present he had accompanied Roberta to several of her sessions, waiting in the outer office for her to finish, and occasionally the three of us would talk when Roberta's time was almost over. Now I called him in and got both their permissions to regress Tom, though it was acknowledged that he would not become my patient. I had worked with couples who had shared earlier lives, and now I was particularly anxious to get Tom's version of things if I could. If Roberta knew he hadn't abandoned her then, perhaps her fear of his abandoning her now would diminish. Tom had a commitment out of town, so an appointment was made for several weeks later.

Roberta returned the following week for her next visit. She regressed effortlessly.

"It's Paris. Summertime. I'm young—no more than twenty-five—and very pretty. All I want to do is have fun, but I can't. My grandmother lives with me. I recognize her. She's Tom."

This was said without surprise. Although what she saw was detailed and vivid, Roberta was not nearly as agitated by this regression as she was by the previous one.

"My grandmother brought me up since both my parents died when I was a little girl, but now I have to take care of her because she's sick and frail. She's demanding, too. Do this, do that. We have no money, so I have to shop, clean, cook, and change my stinky grandmother's clothes because she's always soiling herself."

Finally, she spoke with some vehemence. "It isn't fair! I shouldn't have to do this day after day. A girl's got to have some pleasure in her life." She leaned toward me conspiratorially. "I'm running away. I'm running to my friend Alain's house. He'll take care of me, and he'll show me a good time."

She skipped forward in time, and it is unclear whether her next memories immediately followed this absence from her grandmother's apartment or a later one.

"My grandmother's dead! While I was out drinking, going to cabarets, dancing, making love, she just died. I found her body when I came home. It looks like she starved to death 'cause she was really skinny. None of her neighbors heard her cry out, so it's hard to tell when she died, but it couldn't have been too long ago. She doesn't smell yet, least not any more than she always has. It's bad news, though. Leaves me in an awful pickle. I'm about to have a baby, and I've got no money, not a centime. I'm not even sure who the father is. Alain said he'd give me money if the baby's his, but I had to prove it. Now how am I going to do that until after the baby's born?"

It didn't matter in the end. Roberta saw herself die in child-birth, and her soul floated out of her body. She watched long enough to make sure the baby lived, no matter who the father was. In her life review the overwhelming emotion was guilt.

"I loved my grandmother," she said, "not just because she raised me, but because she was a good woman who wanted only the best for me. But I was too young, too selfish. I put my own needs for freedom and love ahead of her far greater ones. At the very least I could have balanced them, but I ended up abandoning her and—" She stopped abruptly.

"You see the connection," I said, not prompting her but knowing she had indeed related the two regressions.

"Of course! I abandoned her because my husband aban-doned me a thousand years earlier. In Paris he was Tom, my hus-band, who left me to die alone. It was an act of revenge!"

A third regression, which took place a week later, showed us a dif-ferent facet of the same theme of violence and abandonment. This time she was a Pakistani girl living in a small wooden house some five hundred years ago. Her mother had died when she was eleven, and as in Paris, the burden of cooking, cleaning, and other tedious chores fell on her, though in this life she had a father and brother who might have helped her.

"They beat me," she said. "Whenever I did something wrong—if I didn't wash their clothes in time or if they didn't like the food I served—they'd scream at me and hit me, one or the other of them, and sometimes both of them at once."

"Why didn't you leave them?" I asked. "Run away?"

"I needed them for food and shelter." She shivered. "Worse, I was afraid of what my life would be if I went away."

"Anything else?"

"I—I *loved* them."

Her answer surprised me. "Really? Why?"

"Because they couldn't help what they did. After all, our

mother abandoned them by dying. Two of our other siblings died before she did. It was a bleak time, a dark time. There was no law. They were the ones who had to bring home food, which meant that every day there was the possibility of violence, the chance they'd be killed. The illness that struck our mother could have felled any one of us. They had no control over what would happen, no control over nature, over other men, over fate." She shook her head. "To be a man in that time, to have no money and no hope—that was awful."

"So it was because of them, not in spite of them, that you chose to stay," I said.

It was an explanation she had not thought of, but I was sure she would have come to it herself. "Yes."

"What happened next?"

"They stopped beating me. One day they just plain stopped. My father died soon after, but my brother stayed and took me into his household when he married. Eventually, I found a man who loved me, and we moved away. He was a good man, and we led a normal life for that time and place."

"You died happy?"

She sighed. "I died content."

In our present-day review she realized that all three regressions—and particularly the first—explained why she was so afraid that Tom would leave her in his life, but she knew it with her brain, not her heart, and she remained uneasy.

"I'm seeing Tom tomorrow," I said. "Maybe he can help."

He arrived apprehensively. "I'm doing this for Roberta," he said, "to find out about her, not about me."

To prevent distortion I had instructed Roberta not to tell Tom any details of her own past life recollections. I promised him that he would have to undergo only one session unless he chose to come back.

"Not a chance," he said with the wariness of the mystical

that was common to accountants, lawyers, and doctors whose analytical minds beg for precise explanation. I was mildly surprised, therefore, when he reached a deeply relaxed level within a few minutes.

"I'm going to lead you to a past life when you and Roberta were together," I told him, remembering Elizabeth and Pedro from my book *Only Love Is Real* who also remembered sharing past lives. Through them I had discovered the fact of soul mates coming together multiple times and had seen the same phenomenon in other patients.

Almost immediately his back arched as though someone or something had hit him. "I've got to get out of here!" he said desperately.

"Where are you?"

"In a battle. We're surrounded, outflanked. My poor wife! I've left her alone, and I've promised—" His eyes were closed, but he raised his arms as though wielding an axe or a sword. "I'll cut my way out! She *needs* me." With a cry he brought his arms down; then the muscle tension vanished, and his hands lay limply in his lap. "Too late," he whispered. "I'll never see my wife again, never know my child." His last feelings were of guilt and sadness. When I brought him back to the present, he told me he would never leave Roberta again.

When Roberta came for her next session, she was relaxed and smiling; the sunshine had returned. Obviously, she and Tom had spent some time expressing their experiences in the ninth century.

"I now know why he didn't come back to rescue me," she said. "He abandoned me, true, but not because he wanted to, not because I wasn't in his dying thoughts." She laughed. "Well, he's too old now to fight for his country, so I guess I'm safe in this life. With your help, Dr. Weiss, it's clear why I was so afraid he'd leave me, and it's clear that when he says he loves me, he means it. People in love don't go in much for abandonment, do they?"

Roberta was able to let go of her fear of abandonment, her insecurities, and her doubts about Tom. She realized that violence was not necessarily a part of every life and that she was free to choose love instead of fear. This choice was a core theme or pattern in many of her subsequent regressions, and she saw it in the young Pakistani girl who elected to love her father and brother despite their violent natures rather than hate or fear them.

There was one remaining obstacle for Roberta and Tom: their infertility. The loss of her child in the ninth century might explain it, and so might her death during childbirth in nineteenth-century France. But these events had already taken place, she understood, and as with the issue of abandonment, might very well not happen again in this life or future ones.

I decided to try to progress Roberta into the near future so she could fully understand this concept. As always, she quickly reached a peaceful state and was soon observing the course of her life from a higher perspective. "I see two possible life paths," she said, "one with children and the other without."

"Start with 'without.' "

"The one without is dark and narrow, barren. I'm afraid of everything, from insects and snakes to going out of doors. Because we can't have children, Tom has abandoned me, and that adds to my fears. No other man will choose me, and I'm too weak and fearful to exist on my own." She shuddered. "It's awful."

"But with children?" I prompted.

"The world is sunny and wide. Tom is with me, just as he promised. I am happy, fulfilled."

Progressing to this happy life, she was able to completely let go of the fears she had carried over from so many lifetimes: the loss of loved ones and her own death, abandonment, and betrayal. As she was making these connections, her face took on a radiance.

"Where are you?" I asked.

"I'm up very high, higher than the clouds. I'm floating. Floating and watching. It's beautiful here. The air is clear. I can see for miles."

"Are you alone?"

"Yes. Wait—no! Two girls, angelic children, *my* children, are coming to greet me. I can feel their love, feel their joy. Oh, and I love them and I'm joyful!" She paused, watching her future soul. "I recognize them. One is my grandmother, the woman I loved most in the world. She died when I was nine. The other is my mother—not my mother today but the mother of the Pakistani girl I was in a past life five hundred years ago. They're hugging me and I'm hugging them, and I will be with them always."

I have no way of validating Roberta's vision, but I report it accurately. It is her experience, and she really believed this is what would come to pass. It is possible that Roberta and Tom will not be able to conceive and the notion of any children at all is a fantasy—though Roberta and Tom could, of course, adopt children. What is important is that Roberta has full confidence that eventually she will be united with her children, and because of this she is more confident of herself and of her ability to love.

She has made her way from a time of violence to a time of peace; she has made progress toward the point "above the clouds."

Roberta's story demonstrates the harm that violence causes—not just immediately but for future generations, and not just for the victim but for the perpetrator. Those who are violent or who suffer violence may carry their fears and attendant negative emotions ahead to many, many future lifetimes—until they, like Roberta, find love.

Anne's story presents a fascinating contrast to Roberta's, for hers started in the future.

Two days before she came to see me, she awoke from a dream drenched in sweat. It was another of those weird recurrent dreams she had been having; she woke up sweating only if the dream had deep meaning. *The Anne who became the future Anne was determined by her choices,* she heard a voice saying, though she could not see the messenger and did not know if it was male or female. Someone very wise was giving her the message, Anne told me. It seemed to know already what her choices would be, but she had no idea what choices it was talking about. All her life she had acted impulsively and often arbitrarily.

Anne, twenty-four, stocky but not fat, looking like the bespectacled girl who plays the star's best friend in teenage movies, was a graduate student studying architecture up north. Her goal was to design innovative housing complexes, incorporating environmental concerns and allowing the rich and poor to live together. Hers was a vision of people living in harmony in a beautiful setting.

The voice knew of her plan. In a dream she had after we had started working together, it showed her a future where Anne had already designed her project. (It was like a novelist wanting to write a novel and finding out from a messenger that he had already written it in the future.) *Your job is to connect to that future where you've developed your plan, not the one where you have not,* the voice told her. She did not know that I had started progressing patients into the future; she was curious about the meaning of the dream in the present.

She told me an impediment to fulfilling her plan lay in her fear of the limelight. If someone praised her work, she would get anxious. Usually, she would submit her drawings anonymously, even though her professors knew she was the artist. The prospect of winning an award or achieving general recognition filled her with dread. Public success, she knew, would precipitate a panic attack.

Her history indicated no explanation for these reactions in her current life. I was intrigued by her dreams, though, and suggested we look into her future first for more information or clarification. She agreed. While she was in a relaxed trance state, I led her ahead in time to discover what would happen to the housing project.

She watched several future scenarios unfold. In one, there was no project at all. She worked at an architectural firm, but at a mid-level position, drafting the ideas of others. In a second, a housing project was complete, and it incorporated only some of her ideas. It was imperfect, not what she had envisioned. She could see the plaque in the main lobby. Her name was not listed.

The third scenario—triumph! The complex was entirely her design. Her name was first on the architectural drawings and on the plaque. Yet when she reported it, she did not seem happy. (There were several other possible scenarios as well, but not as distinct as these three.)

"It's the fear," she said when I brought her back. "The fear of recognition, the fear of success. I realize I can go any of the ways, but the third seems the most terrifying. *I don't want my name on that plaque.*"

In fact, the plaque was not a sign of ego; it was a symbol representing the absence of fears and of her panic attacks. Her name would not go on it as long as she was afraid. I knew we would have to look into her past for the healing to take place.

In her first regression Anne was a boy in an ancient horse-riding culture of central Asia. The chief of her nomadic village had a son who was two years older than Anne but did not possess Anne's skill at horseback riding, at archery, or with a saber. "He doesn't like me," Anne reported simply. The other boy was being groomed to be his father's successor, and it infuriated the old man to see his son continually bested. Anne was oblivious to the effects of her success, yet more and more the chieftain's son was humiliated by Anne's victories.

"There was a riding contest for all the young men in the village," Anne said. "It was one I determined to win, and I did. The entire town, women and men, feted me for my achievement. I drank too much and lay down in a field outside the village to sleep. The chieftain's son snuck up silently and slit my throat. I did not die quickly. I watched my wine-red blood flow out."

In our discussion after I led her back, Anne told me she had not begun to apprehend the mortal danger her successes created. "Of course!" she exclaimed. "Sitting here with you now it's easy to link outward success with great physical harm. No wonder I'm afraid."

She could see the pattern of success creating danger in a kaleidoscopic string of images of past lives during her next regression. In one she was a talented musician, a man ruined by his rival who stole Anne's music and presented it as his own. In another she was a girl in a Near Eastern kingdom some two thousand years ago. Upper-class boys of her age were taught arcane secrets and rituals forbidden to girls, but Anne spied on the restricted classes and learned what they did. One day, being taunted by the boys, she blurted out one of the secrets. "You see," she said, "I know just as much as you do." She paid for her arrogance with her life. She was reported, jailed, and soon killed because death was the punishment for breaking the taboo.

As we processed these experiences, Anne was able to pinpoint the equations. Success meant violence. Self-exposure meant punishment. Pride meant death. Gradually, with more therapy, she was able to realize that her panic at being in the limelight was a consequence of past life experiences, not something she had to fear in her present or future lives. With difficulty, for her terror went deep, she was able to relinquish her fears. She began to sign her class drawings, and she built a scale model of her building complex, winning a prize for "Most Innovative Design." She could not go so far as to give an acceptance speech, she admitted, but the prize, a silver plaque, stands on her mantel.

We both have an idea of the futures that Anne will find herself in. Indeed, *the Anne who will become the future Anne will be determined by her choices.* She no longer sweats when the Master comes back to remind her.

CHAPTER 8

Bruce:
Relationships

WHEN WE ARE IN HUMAN FORM, even though our ultimate goal is to merge with the spirit, the one soul, interaction with others physically, emotionally, and spiritually lies at the core of our life. How we handle this plays a large part in determining our future.

A woman I know who spent her adult life in an ashram was a spiritual person, but she complained to me that she couldn't meditate at all. In one of my own meditations I understood why. She needed to go out into the world, to be in many relationships, to experience loss and grief, joy and love. For all her spirituality, she had vital lessons to learn.

We all have many different types of relationships: one-on-one; with our families and loved ones; with the people we work with—bosses, colleagues, and other employees; with our friends; and with teachers and students. Across our many lives their bodies may change and the relationships with them may change, but we are still learning the lesson of the importance of relationships, because we come around again and again with the same soul.

Maybe your mother has been pushing your buttons for many

lifetimes. Maybe, in different lifetimes, you've been her mother, and maybe you've been in other relationships with her that are not mother and child. Eventually, we must heal all our relationships, and we must use all our skills to do this, especially empathy, compassion, nonviolence, and love. Communication is the key to every relationship. Love and openness are vital to the process, but so is safety, for if it's not safe to communicate, you won't.

How do you make the environment for communication safe? By knowing first of all that there are many ways of communicating—words, thoughts, body language, expression in the eyes and face, touch—and that each must be attended to. You should also understand that the soul with whom you have a relationship may have been important to you in the past during many lifetimes and over many centuries, and may be important in future centuries as well.

A recent patient of mine was horrified to think that a codependent relationship she had with an abusive man, one she had just managed to escape, was not over; she realized that the man might return to her in a future life. "How can I prevent it?" she asked. "I don't want him back."

The answer is to make sure there are no hooks in you that will pull him back—no anger, no violence, nothing negative at all. If you can leave a relationship with love, empathy, and compassion, without any thoughts of revenge, hatred, or fear, that is how you let go.

You can choose to no longer have a relationship with that person or persons. You can interact only with those you feel a kinship to, only with those whom, in its broadest definition, you love. In future lives you will be together with many of your loved ones, your soul mates, because you are functioning as a family of souls. Others will have to catch up, to learn the lessons you have mastered, before they, too, can join your community of souls.

* * *

One of the most moving examples of relationships in action involved Bruce who came to me last year in terrible shape. He was suffering, he told me, from symptoms of chronic anxiety: sleeplessness, heart palpitations, sudden rages, and occasional alcoholic binges. He was a nondescript man with wet eyes, a wet handshake, and closely cropped brown hair that hid incipient baldness. His speech retained cadences of the Midwest—he was from Milwaukee—but he had lived in Miami for two years with Frank, a producer fifteen years his senior (Bruce was thirty-five) who was connected with one of our regional theaters. Frank had once had a blazing career, but a series of flops had reduced his reputation and his income, forcing him to move from a mansion in Los Angeles to a humble house in Coral Gables. It changed him from a witty, contented man to a sour soul who took much of his depression out on Bruce through sarcasm and public humiliation. Of late they had taken to fighting with each other both privately and publicly, though neither wanted to end the relationship.

Bruce was a costume designer. The two had met when Frank hired him for a production. They had entered a physical relationship quickly. Both men preferred to keep it clandestine and so lived apart in Los Angeles, sharing lodging only when they moved to Miami.

When I asked Bruce why he stayed since Frank had become so difficult, he merely shrugged and said, "With it all, I love him."

"Yes, but moving out doesn't mean you'd have to stop seeing each other. It might loosen Frank's hold on you," I said. "And it might ease some of your anxiety. How does he humiliate you?"

"By calling me a faggot or his mistress in front of our friends and by making me do things I don't like—sexual things—in private."

"You don't fight back?"

"Sometimes. More these last few months. And the anger

comes out in other ways, too. But most of the time I keep it inside, hidden. Particularly in bed."

"You say it comes out in other ways—when you drink, for instance? Inappropriately, I presume."

"I get mad at bartenders and whores."

"Male whores?"

"Of course." A slight shudder showed what he thought of the
idea of sleeping with women.

"Do you frequent them often?"

"No. From time to time."

"Why?"

"When I get tired of Frank hurting me and want to hurt
someone back."

"Physically hurt them?"

Another shudder. "No. I make them do some of the things
I'm forced to do with Frank."

A strange kind of revenge, I thought. "Could you give them
up?" I asked. "Redirect your anger toward the person who pro-
voked it?"

He was quiet for a moment. Then he said, "I'm not sure I
could show Frank the real depth of my anger. It's too dangerous.
But I've given up the whores."

"It's a start," I said. "Good for you."

His wet eyes overflowed, and he bowed his head. "No, bad
for me."

"Why? It seems—"

He stopped me. "I have AIDS. I don't want to infect anyone
with it."

His overall health had been declining for some months, he
told me. He had a gastric ulcer, and the birthmark on his abdomen had recently and inexplicably begun to bleed. Panicked,
he had it biopsied, but no cancer was found and he was briefly relieved. Still, the large scar that was left at the site would from time
to time turn beet red and ooze a drop or two of blood. This led

him to his internist, who diagnosed AIDS. "More a confirmation of my fears than a diagnosis," he said. Tests were taken. The diagnosis was verified two weeks ago. Because of it, he made an appointment with me.

I could help him with his anxiety and his relationship with Frank, I said, but I could not cure him of the disease, though "cocktails" were now in wide use that would slow down its progress and add years to his life.

His expression was profoundly sad. "Extra years are no good unless I can get my life together."

"Then let me ask: Do your parents know you're homosexual?"

"They do now. I kept it from them as long as I could—I even made up a California girlfriend I'd write them about—but when Frank and I moved here and started living together, they found out."

"Their reaction?"

"Shock. Denial. Believe it or not: 'Wasn't there some medicine I could take?' I think they're more concerned about their friends knowing than anything else. After all, it's the Midwest, and they're about a century behind the rest of the country." He put his hand to his forehead in a theatrical gesture. " 'The shame of it!' "

I laughed despite myself.

"They're good people, loving people—just ignorant on this subject," he went on. "When I go home to visit, they greet me with love and respect. It's my brother who's the problem."

"Your brother?"

"I guess I forgot to mention him. Yes, Ben's a Milwaukee big shot. Senior vice president at Aetna. Lots of money, lots of friends, lots of clout. The Republicans have dangled the word *congressman* before his eyes, and he's been salivating after it like a dog at the track."

"And a gay brother—?"

He shrugged. "Good-bye Washington. He came to see me about a year ago and actually asked me to change my name. I told him to go fuck himself. He persisted: 'It might be good if you disappeared for a while. At least don't tell anybody you're my brother.' Well, that got me. How dare he! I'm just as good as he is—better—even though my lover's a man. I went after him. My last sight of him was his sorry ass running down Coral Way."

If this was one of his sudden rages, it seemed to me justified. I told him so.

"True, but like when I'm angry at Frank, when I think of Ben's attitude, I explode—wherever I am and against whomever I'm with. Ben is just a half-assed, greedy, glorified insurance salesman. I pity him, and it's ridiculous that I want to kill him. I *am* the better man, and better men don't hold a grudge—or a dozen of them."

His rages did seem too violent to be explained solely by the circumstances of his life. And while his anxiety was natural, given the diagnosis of AIDS, I wondered if it was always so severe that, like now, it affected his life.

"Yes," he answered when I asked about it. "Even in school when I had every reason to be happy—good student, loving parents, that sort of thing—I always felt a sense of dread. Now that I have something real to dread, it has gotten worse, but not that much worse."

"Maybe it comes from something that happened in your past," I said.

"My childhood? No. As I just told you, it was extremely normal."

"Not your childhood," I said, "your distant past."

He leaned forward. "Explain."

I did explain, and he agreed to a regression. Surprisingly, because I thought Bruce would be leery of hypnosis, not wanting to allow himself to become too vulnerable, he could go under more deeply than all but a few of my patients, and what he remembered was vivid.

"I am in ancient Egypt. It is during the reign of the great Pharaoh whose ambition is to build temples and palaces proclaiming his might and his magnificence. There have been temples built before, but these are to be grander than anything ever attempted. I am an engineer, and the Pharaoh has chosen me to work on two projects: the creation of a sanctuary and the erection of connecting colonnades.

"I have actually met with the Pharaoh himself; it was there he described his plans. It is of course an incalculable honor to be selected, and if I succeed, anything of my asking shall be mine for the rest of my life. When I told him I would need five hundred laborers and slaves, he offered a thousand. No expense is to be spared, no death in service of the ultimate goal regretted. The buildings are to sanctify this supreme divinity and must reflect his supremacy.

"Still, the Pharaoh has issued stringent commands. The sanctuary is to be completed in seven years, the colonnades three years later. Only the finest marble can be used, only the strongest stones. We are to make sure that when it is completed, the result will proclaim his glory for all eternity.

"The task is difficult. There are the practical problems of transporting the stones and the marble, to say nothing of having adequate water on hand, and wood for the rails on which to raise the stones. The weather, even in the winter, is blazing hot. Sand- and windstorms are persistent hazards. Architects and engineers of equal talent, or so the Pharaoh believes, will be designing and building other temples, other colonnades. We will no doubt be in competition with one another for what necessarily must be limited supplies, even given the Pharaoh's wealth.

"And there is one more impediment. The Pharaoh has a cousin. I've met the man, a meddler, a sycophant, an egomaniac with no talent and less taste. He is the overseer of the entire project. I and all the other architects and engineers are to obey him. His word is the Pharaoh's word and thus is law. I am frightened of him. He could wreck everything."

Indeed, Bruce paled as he spoke of the overseer. The man continued to exert his power even in the stillness of my office. I was struck by the formality of Bruce's language, quite different from the colloquial speech he used ordinarily. When I later asked him if he had ever been to Egypt, he assured me he hadn't. History and travel to historic sites did not appeal to him.

I led him forward in this past life.

"My worries are confirmed," Bruce continued. "He meddles in everything. He seems to dislike me in particular. Perhaps he can sense my aversion to him, though I forbear to express it. At any rate he is at my side nearly every day, offering ludicrous suggestions, countermanding my orders, complaining that my comrades and I are working too slowly, although it is he who stands in the way of progress. Given the time strictures laid down by the Pharaoh, this increases the pressure on me to a point where I am sure I will explode. Every day means a battle with myself to stay calm in the face of demands and his taunts when I can't satisfy them.

"About a year after work started, the scoundrel insists that the sanctuary be placed next to a different temple rather than by the foremost temple. When I remind him that this is directly contrary to the Pharaoh's orders, he calls me a fool in front of my colleagues and starts to walk off.

"What I fear comes to pass: I explode. I tell him he's the fool, that he's nothing but an idiot and looks the part, that he is as stupid as the stones surrounding him. 'Let's take this matter to the Pharaoh,' I say. 'He will decide who should have final authority.'

"The Pharaoh's cousin retaliates in the worst way possible. Rather than go with me to the palace, he enlists a rival of mine, another engineer, to poison the wine I drink at dinner. I fall sick immediately; the pain is excruciating, and I am put to bed. That night one of the guards sneaks into my tent and stabs me in the stomach. I die instantly. My last sight is of the Pharaoh's wretched cousin standing outside my tent, laughing."

I brought him back; he was visibly shaken. "Can you express what you're feeling?" I asked.

"The . . . the place on my stomach where I was stabbed," he stammered. "It's the same place where I have the scar tissue from the biopsy, the wound that bleeds from time to time for no apparent reason."

"Anything else?"

He was in an ecstasy of revelation. "The overseer, the man who tormented me in Egypt during that past life, he's my brother in this one."

Anger, as he had admitted, was a negative factor in his present life. It was at its most virulent when he was confronting or was confronted by his brother Ben who, after all, had asked Bruce to give up his identity, to become invisible.

I was as anxious as he to revisit another past life. Again, it was in ancient Egypt, at another time.

"I'm a priest, a healer, one of a very few employed by the rich and powerful. Our medicine is arcane, not the usual herbs and lotions that lay doctors use. My healing method involves the use of what we priests call energy rods. When the rods are turned in precisely the right way, they emit healing sound vibrations and light frequencies. Their use is not random. There is a prescribed sequence of light and sound, an intricate order and pattern to how the rods are aimed at portions of the body. The art is secret. It involves energy and light and their accumulation, storage, and transfer."

"Where do you practice this medicine?" I asked.

His eyes glittered. "In secret chambers within the healing temples. Only a few priests know of their location. Even those who do menial work in the temples do not know of them, so masterfully are they hidden."

"And you are able to work wonders?"

"Exactly! We have cured many diseases." He leaned forward. "And we are able to regenerate organs and limbs lost in battle."

"Through the use of the rods?"

"The rods. Yes."

"Amazing."

I had read about healing techniques and medicine in ancient cultures, and while I had never read about the rods that Bruce described, I did know that Egyptian doctors claimed they could regenerate limbs and organs, and that they had apparently accomplished wonders in curing blood diseases, immune diseases, and diseases of the skin and brain. There is, in fact, an inner chamber in one of the Luxor temples that was used as a medical room; its walls are covered with paintings that show the doctors at work in these fields.

I next saw Bruce a month later. In the interim he had developed pneumonia, a common side effect of AIDS, and had to be hospitalized. When he returned, his face was very white and he seemed exhausted, though when I volunteered to put off our sessions, he insisted we go on.

"They're doing healing things for me," he said. "I can't explain precisely why, but I feel I'm on the edge of something vitally important. It's essential I understand what it is before I die."

Rather than have him go back again, although it would have been valuable, I decided to see if I could use the mind-body connection to alleviate his physical symptoms. "I want to try an experiment," I told him. "Are you up for it?"

"Sure. Anything."

"Then I want you to switch roles in your mind. You are an Egyptian patient receiving light and sound energy, and I want you to transfer that energy into your present body and mind."

This was unorthodox, granted, but I did it because he was HIV positive and was suffering pain at the site of the biopsy.

"Who should your doctor be?" I asked.

"Frank," he answered immediately. "We've had our differences, but underneath it all, he still loves me."

"Frank is with you in your Egyptian life," I said. "He's a priest-healer; he knows the arcane sciences. Let him apply his knowledge to you."

Bruce closed his eyes and leaned back in his chair. I could see his facial muscles relax, and a bit of color returned to his cheeks. "It's working. I feel better."

"Excellent. Your doctor understands the use of the rods; he knows the patterns and the order of light and sound. This is the highest level of healing. Be grateful for it."

"I am," he whispered. "Oh, I am!"

The rest of the session was spent in silence. When Bruce left, I told him to meditate at home. "The light and the healing will be with you there. It needn't be confined to this office."

He came back not only feeling healthier but with insights. "My brother was with me in both past lives," he said. "He was the overseer in the first, but in the second he was with me as another priest-healer. And when you asked me to go back to that life and be the patient, it was Ben who turned out to be the healer of me, not Frank."

"I'm sure that's right. Now put yourself in Ben's place in both lifetimes. Project yourself into his body and his perspective."

He concentrated for several minutes, frowning with the effort. Then his eyes opened, and his smile was incandescent. "He's jealous of me! Both in the past life and this one. Even though he's the powerful one, the administrator or the politician, he's jealous. It's his own suffering that makes him so cruel."

Bruce explained that although his brother was an Egyptian noble and administrator, he nevertheless resented Bruce's talent and skills, which he did not possess nor could he ever learn. He was raised in an environment of absolute privilege and power, and when Bruce lashed out at him in public, he had to avenge the humiliation.

"Thus the poison," Bruce said. "The knife thrust was extra. It was powered by anger, jealousy, and shame."

He was obviously undergoing an intense empathic experience. I have rarely seen a patient so moved. "What about your present life? What's your brother jealous of now?"

The answer came quickly: "My parents' love. Maybe because I was the more fragile child, they paid more attention to me than him—'Ben's so strong, he can get along by himself'—and to him that meant they loved me more, though I'm not sure that's true. *This* is the revelation. I wish I had known it sooner."

I asked the psychiatrist's core question: "How does it make you feel?"

"Forgiving. Loving. He's not the powerful other. He's just like me, a mixture of strength and weakness. It's glorious!"

"Do you think he could feel the same way?"

"Of course. If I can, he can, for we are the same. My second life in Egypt taught me that."

"Can you teach him?"

"I can try."

As I write this, Bruce has made enormous progress. His abdominal wound has healed; it never turns red or seeps blood. His ulcer is similarly healed. He and Frank have resolved their sexual issues, and they have stopped fighting, though they still squabble. I think they both enjoy it. Through his past life and spiritual experiences he has lost his fear of death. He does not see his brother as all-powerful and realizes some of this feeling came from his own projections onto Ben. Of all the lessons his regression has taught him, the most powerful, he thinks, is that relationships are in their profoundest sense between equals, and if he can laud the strengths of the other and forgive the weaknesses—for they are ours as well—then love will follow. He and his brother see each other often and communicate daily.

"He has turned my being gay into a political plus," Bruce told me with a grin. "Now he's a 'liberal Republican.' In Wisconsin you can't do better."

In one of our last sessions he told me that when he was the Egyptian priest-healer, he sometimes oversaw the healing ceremonies attendant to the application of the rods. In these ceremonies he connected the power of the healing energies, light and sound, which in Egyptian times were believed to connect to the power of the divinities but are now, he knows, attributes of the one god or the One. Bruce knows that he is and always has been immortal, that all of us are eternally interconnected, and that we are forever embraced by love.

CHAPTER 9

Patrick:
Security

WE HEAR THE WORD *security* every day. Financial security, Social Security, national security—all these are important. But here we are discussing a more profound security, security of *self:* emotional security, psychic security, security that enables us to interact fully with our families, our lovers, our friends, our society, our civilization.

It springs from self-love, from understanding yourself as a soul, and from realizing you were present in past lives and will exist in future lives throughout all time. Real security comes from the knowledge that you are immortal, that you are eternal, and that you can never be harmed.

I've treated very wealthy people who are miserable and have no sense of security at all, though their creature comforts are assured throughout their present lives. Security doesn't come from possessions. You can't bring your material things into the next life, but you can bring your deeds, your actions, and your growth—what you have learned and how you are progressing as a spiritual human being. It is also possible that you can take some of your talents. I have the idea that Mozart was an accomplished musician in an earlier life, which accounts for his precocity as a child in the eighteenth century.

Security and self-esteem are interrelated, and self-esteem is sometimes difficult to achieve, though without it self-love isn't possible. Many of us incorporate the concept taught (usually unconsciously) by our parents, teachers, friends, or communities that we are deficient in some way, not up to the mark. If we can let go of the negatives, we can gain self-love. The religious traditions that say "love everybody else" miss the point. Self-love is the basis for love of others. It is where real charity begins. When you love yourself, it will spill over; when you don't love yourself, your energy will consciously or unconsciously be focused on finding it, and you won't have time for anybody else.

Self-love isn't selfish; it's healthy self-esteem. The egotist, the braggart, the self-promoter, the diva, and the salesman—those who come across as self-loving in order to sell themselves or their products—are often insecure at heart. The man I once thought was the most put-together person I knew, a model of public self-assurance and self-promotion, told me in a moment of mutual confidence that he played a game called "dodge the bus," which meant he stood at a dangerous street corner and tried to see how close he could come to being hit.

"What if you were killed?" I asked, flabbergasted.

"Then the world would be rid of a worthless thing," he answered.

True self-love doesn't need to be broadcast or publicly displayed. It is an inner state, a feeling, a strength, a happiness; it is security. Remember, souls are part of the One, which is love. We all have souls. We are always loved. We can always love in return.

When Patrick entered my office for the first time, he looked like a scruffy adolescent—hair tousled, wispy beard, jeans and Marlins jacket that needed a wash, untied Adidas sneakers and filthy fingernails—but he was actually thirty-one. A cadaverously thin young man with rheumy eyes that he averted and a limp handshake, this was a man whose self-esteem was as low as that of anyone I've ever encountered.

We established his age, residence (Miami), that he was still living with his parents, profession (accountant for a fledgling dot-com company), and the fact that he was an only child and single—"a virgin," he told me with a flush of shame.

"Who recommended me?" I asked.

"My parents."

"Do I know them?"

"No. There is no way you would. My father works in the shipping office of a factory, and my mom is a saleslady at Kmart. Not the sort of people you hobnob with."

The last was said hostilely. I let it pass but thought they must love their son deeply to spend the money for his therapy. "Then how did they find out about me?"

"They heard you on a TV show and immediately it was 'That's the man for Patrick.'"

"Why?"

"Because I'm into science fiction—or was."

"And they think past life regression is science fiction?" I looked at him closely. "Do you?"

A shrug. Silence. I pressed on: "You said you were into science fiction. When was that?"

"When I was a kid."

"But you're not anymore?"

"Oh, I guess I am. But I'm too old for it."

Remarkable. Many of my adult friends read science fiction and have lent me books by writers I admire: Verne, Wells, Lem, Bradbury. I was particularly interested in them now since they had extraordinary visions of the future. "What's 'too old'?"

"Twelve."

He said it with such assurance that I knew an event had happened when he was that age which had somehow scarred him. "You were too old when you reached twelve? Other people read science fiction until they're ninety."

Another shrug. *Granted.* "Who said you were too old?"

"My dad. He took my books and sold them to a secondhand bookstore. He said it was time for me to prepare for what I'd do when I was grown up."

"And science fiction would interfere with that?"

"I was a dreamer, he said, living on Mars. It was time to come back to Earth."

"Was he right?"

"I suppose so." Patrick leaned forward and at last his voice became animated. "But I'll tell you, Dr. Weiss. It was a lot better living on Mars than it is on Earth."

Then how unhappy his life on Earth must be.

"What do you think of the probes of Mars now?" I asked. "Have you seen the pictures?"

"Have I! And that's just the beginning. In ten years there'll be humans on Mars, colonies of them."

"Will you be there?"

The light went out of it as though I'd switched it off. "Nah."

"Because you're not allowed to?"

"Because others will have gotten there first." He put his hands together and brought them in front of his eyes, as though to blot out my face. "They wouldn't want me with them."

Again I felt his unhappiness. "Why?"

"Because I don't belong. Because I never belong."

"Where do you belong?"

"Alone in the sky."

"How do you know?"

"That's what the books told me."

"The science fiction books?"

"Right. Only to me they didn't seem like fiction—they were glimpses of the future. I'd be in this spaceship or even flying on my own; it was easy. I didn't like the books where there were wars and such. I didn't like monsters or super weapons. Just the books about traveling to other planets or the stars."

I could picture him self-imprisoned in his room, reading,

while his parents fretted below, wondering what to do with their peculiar child.

"Even when you stopped reading," I said, "when you tried to do what your father wanted, tried to fit in, you were alone."

He looked at me as though I were a magician. "Yes. When I tried to talk about the sky or about other planets or space travel, the kids didn't seem interested. But it was all I knew about, all I *cared* about. I could go where others couldn't, and they didn't want to hear about it. The kids thought I was crazy, all except Donnie who was my friend. He was the only boy I felt comfortable with, but then his parents moved away and he went with them."

"Which left you completely alone."

"The thing is, I began to think there was something wrong with me. I was different, I knew that, but *why?* I felt all-powerful, but it turns out I had no power at all. My dad told me science fiction was for kids, but if that was so, why didn't kids read it? I gave it up like he wanted, but my life felt empty. It wasn't fun anymore. I had no place to go, no place to hide. Since nobody paid attention to me, nobody *listened,* I couldn't trust myself. I like numbers—there's a mathematics to space—so I became an accountant. An *accountant!* Is there anything more normal? Is there anything more dull? I felt completely empty, hopeless."

Patrick's long speech was accompanied by a series of facial expressions—sadness, anger, despair, blankness—that were the physical signs of his inner turmoil.

"You shouldn't listen to others so much," I said quietly. "Follow your intuition. There's nothing wrong with being a loner—and, anyway, just as you found Donnie, you'll find others, men and women, who'll think as you do."

He shrugged, then turned his head away. I could sense he was fighting back tears.

"What's the matter?" I asked.

"You told me I shouldn't listen to others."

"Yes. It's good advice."

"That's just the trouble. It isn't."

"I don't understand."

Now he looked at me, and his answer was an anguished wail: "I feel hopeless, desperate, despairing. If I don't listen to others, then I'll have to listen to myself!"

Memories of past lives came easily to him under hypnosis. "I'm a male," he said, "but not exactly a man, not exactly human."

I tried to hide my amazement, but I'm afraid my voice might have cracked. "What time period are you talking about?"

"Sixty thousand years ago."

"Sixty thou—" I stared at him, trying to see if the hypnosis hadn't worked and he was putting me on. No. His eyes were closed, his breathing regular. "Go on," I managed to say.

"I was born on another planet. It had no name. Maybe it existed in a different planetary system or a different dimension. Anyway, I'm part of a migration from my planet to Earth. When we arrive, others greet us, descendants of beings from earlier migrations from different star systems. They're mixed among an evolving subspecies, human beings. We must stay on Earth with them because our planet is dying and this one is new. True, we needn't have physically come here. Our souls could have been reincarnated into the humans around us or into the beings from other worlds. But we are a proud people. Our technology is advanced—we have traveled vast distances—our culture is sophisticated, and our intelligence is acute. We want to preserve our knowledge and our accomplishments. We want to join the others and through reincarnation aid the evolution of these new human people."

The Patrick in my office had a high voice as though it had not fully matured. It was appropriate to his personality. Now, however, his tone was resonant, and the words flowed with great authority. I was spellbound by his vision, one unlike any I had ever encountered.

"Our bodies are not too different from the humans', but our minds are far superior. The atmosphere on Earth is much like the one surrounding our old planet, which is why we chose this location as our destination, but the air here is pure and clear. In all other respects, too, the Earth is far more beautiful than the place from which we came. There are trees and grass and water, rivers and oceans, and flowers, birds, and fish of every color. I am content here—no, more than content. Happier than I've ever been. My job is to supervise the storage of artifacts and written knowledge, and I have found the ideal place: natural chambers deep under the Earth's surface. By the time humans have reached a level where they can understand what we have hidden, they will be able to find it."

Later, when I had a chance to ponder what he was saying, several ideas that I had formed before I met him seemed verified. Souls are the same, I believed, whether they come from different dimensions or galaxies or from Earth. New arrivals to our world quickly enter the reincarnation cycle and then tend to incarnate here, in part because they have created karmic debts and obligations, in part because their mission is to assist in the evolution of the human race. Souls can enter earthly bodies as easily as any "alien" body. Patrick's soul chose to stay in this "paradise" that his people had chosen to inhabit.

With my urging, Patrick took me further ahead in this past life. "I have found a cliff where the ocean meets the sky, and I have built a house there of stone and wood. My huge task is complete; the artifacts and documents are safely stored. I am free to enjoy the beauty around me, to bask in the scented air. I am considered wise, and many of my own race, as well as humans, come to me for advice, which I am happy to give. Eventually I die, but long ago my people learned to detach their souls from their physical bodies at the proper moment so they can move with ease to levels of higher consciousness. This I do, but I am able to continue communication with many of my people still in their bodies in their new home, the planet Earth."

Indeed, he seemed transported, floating between two realms, in two levels of consciousness. "The distinction between God and humans is minor," he said. "One of the pieces of knowledge that remain hidden where I have had it stored is how to master the art of separating consciousness from the physical vehicle. Someday soon your culture will learn how to do that, too. When that happens, you will find that the separating awareness can assume other, less 'solid' bodies as it wishes. From that vantage it can influence other entities in their physical forms. To the receiving entity this influence will seem divine, angelic, godlike. But it is really an advanced form of the very same consciousness possessed by the receiver."

To hear such profound thoughts from a young man who seemed at first meeting callow and unformed was thrilling. And what he said next was, to me, beautiful.

"My world is ancient and yours is very young, yet the difference is as nothing in the scope of time. Time is like a breath out and a breath in by a cosmic god. The out-breath is the creation of stars, planets, galaxies, and universes. The in-breath brings them all back into one incredibly small and dense point of dust in the god's lungs. The respiration of time, in and out, occurring in an endless number of cycles, hints at the nature of eternity."

Patrick fell silent, and I, much moved, considered his words. My own studies, I felt, had been enhanced. I had been shown, as Patrick said, a glimpse of "the nature of eternity," and it seemed to me exquisite. I understood his attraction to science fiction, his love for the sky, and the wish for the ability to travel to the stars. When he awakened, I asked him if he believed that what he had witnessed was merely an extension of the books he had loved as a child.

"No," he said quickly. "I never imagined anything like what I saw just now, and neither did the writers of the books. My experience was very real. I imagined nothing."

His reaction seemed authentic and sparked in him a wave of ideas.

"What if black holes are actually part of the cosmic in-breath?" he wondered aloud. "What if angels and masters and spiritual guides are somehow linked to ancient and highly advanced alien civilizations?"

Far out, I thought. Over the edge. But that's what I had thought when Catherine began her regressions and when Victoria told me she had seen me in Jerusalem. Besides, what I thought didn't matter. I could see a new light in Patrick's eyes, the spark of his passion returning after more than twenty years. Further therapy would bring him closer to his spiritual path, I knew. It would bring him to it by renewing his passion for life, his joy and his hope.

As therapy progressed, Patrick was able to remember three additional past lives:

1. As an indigenous inhabitant of either Central America or the northern part of South America nine centuries ago, he was renowned as a mathematician and an astronomer, living alone but revered and honored to an old age. His experience sixty thousand years ago influenced this lifetime, he realized, for he was curious about the configuration of the stars and the meaning of meteors.

2. In the early eighteenth century he was a kabbalistic Jewish rabbi, a scholar living in a small town outside Krakow, Poland. There he was able to combine his mystical studies with a practical family life. He had much to teach, had a wife and many children, and was comfortable and accepted by the townsfolk and his culture. He did not feel like an "alien" as he often did in this current life.

3. He was a Buddhist monk living in a cold and barren
part of China in the fourteenth century. There he was
well accepted in the community of religious thinkers
and was able to combine periods of meditation and
introspection with an active farming life. He was a
master of energy manipulation and flow, particularly the
energy centers and channels within the body. When he
was back in the present, he understood how similar his
work was to the practice of acupuncture. As he relived
this Chinese lifetime, he sensed his immediate transcendence beyond the physical and mortal to a place in
another realm in a parallel universe. Many of these
concepts were similar to the knowledge and wisdom he
would acquire several centuries later as the kabbalistic
rabbi; he could see the connection immediately as we
reviewed this Buddhist life in my office. Either the cultures had communicated at some time in the past, he
surmised, or the knowledge was indeed universal and
could be tapped into independently by anyone wishing
to use his or her intelligence in the pursuit of what lay
beyond the perceptible world.

By this time Patrick felt comfortable with me and, as he put it,
"enjoyed my sessions as much as I enjoyed reading science fiction." But he still had difficulty in the Miami outside my office.
While he was less influenced by the values and opinions of other
people, particularly his father, he still felt insecure in the presence
of women and all strangers. "Now instead of feeling despairing,"
he said, "I just feel lonely. My thoughts are nice to go to sleep
with, but I'd be happier if a woman's body was alongside me to
keep them company." He closed his eyes. "Maybe in a future life,"
he said wistfully.

"Maybe," I said. "Would you like to try to find out?"

* * *

"My name is Maddie," Patrick said. "Women aren't usually asked to participate in high-level astronomical research, but my grades were so superior to my male counterparts' and my work so good at the space center that they couldn't keep me away—I'd have sued them."

Some things don't change, I thought. Sexism in the future doesn't sound very different from sexism in the present. I liked Maddie immediately. She was obviously a fierce and tough advocate for herself, a good progression for Patrick.

"What year is it?" I asked.

"Year twenty-two fifty-four," she answered immediately. "Month May, day Thursday, time ten-seventeen P.M."

"How old are you?"

"Thirty-one"—the age Patrick was in this life.

"Where are you speaking from?"

"The observatory, of course. Here I am, surrounded by my computers, my 'scopes, my listening devices. I've been here since nine this morning—my usual hours—and I couldn't be happier."

"What specifically are you working on?"

She sighed. "I suppose it's all right to tell. The press got hold of the story a few weeks ago and have been making fun of it ever since. My friends laugh at me, too, but I assure you it's dead serious."

"I have no doubt of it," I said gravely.

"We're studying the origin, structure, and occasional demise of alien civilizations."

I confess to being stunned. If this was fantasy, it was appropriate for Patrick, a direct continuation of his childhood reading. But if it was real, and if his life sixty thousand years ago was real, then how marvelous that at this future point in time he could study the roots of his past.

"Where does your information come from?"

Maddie seemed pleased by the question, adopting a professorial tone familiar to me from my college days. "Simply put—and what we do is by no means simple—we've been utilizing data from space probes to 'listen' to the messages from other planets in other galaxies. What we learn from them is then combined with information gathered from the sixteen space stations we've orbited throughout the solar system, and by now we have a pretty good idea of the landscape. It seems there are dozens of such civilizations, such societies. Most are too far away for us to make anything but the most rudimentary contacts—signals sent from them to us and from us to them that tell both societies that we *exist*. But with others, the closer ones, those that have the technology to accomplish it—well, it seems we'll be having some visits pretty soon."

"Will they visit us, or will we visit them?"

"Oh, they'll come to us. We're not nearly advanced enough in space travel. We've barely been able to get beyond our own solar system." She paused, eyes bright. "But when they do come and we can show them to the world, think of the increases in government funding!"

"You'll be there to see it," I said.

"You bet! And the press and my friends who laughed at us. They'll be eating crow."

Maddie was hazy about family, friends, and personal relationships. When I asked about them, she changed the subject back to her work. Clearly, this was the part of his future life which inspired Patrick, and as always I did not press the patient to go where he was reluctant to investigate.

I was about to ask him for more details about Maddie's research when his awareness shifted, and he left that lifetime to come back to the current one; still hypnotized, he viewed it from a higher perspective.

"For the past three years I'd been thinking of taking an astronomy course at the University of Miami. I'd audit it if they wouldn't accept me as a full-time student. But I always postponed it—too shy to ask, I guess. But now I see I'm meant to take the course. It is the next step in preparation for my future life and work." He took a breath, then said slowly and calmly, "It's the destiny I've been searching for."

After he left, I wrote a note on the concepts of destiny and free will that are so important to my work: "Patrick would be choosing to take the astronomy course, yet it would also be his destiny. The two are strongly linked. The correct application of our free will could carry us along the path of our destiny. On the other hand, free choices that are not correct could carry us away from our destiny, delaying our spiritual progress and complicating our lives. It's much easier to make correct choices if we can glimpse our future, whether in this life or in lives to come."

Seeing his future life certainly crystallized Patrick's decision to take the astronomy course. He enrolled at the next opportunity.

Patrick soon received confirmation that he was indeed on the path of his true destiny. During the second semester of his astronomy course, he called me. By that time we had long finished his therapy, and I hadn't heard from him since his discharge. "I need to see you," he said.

Uh-oh. We made a date, and I wondered what could possibly have happened. Patrick had been transformed from a man with debilitating insecurities to one who seemed at peace with himself and with his limitations. From his long silence I assumed he was getting along well, but maybe something had thrown him back into his former disquiet.

To the contrary, he bounded into my office like an over-zealous puppy and clasped my hand in a firm grip. Whereas he used to avoid my eyes, now he looked into them with a steady gaze.

"What's up?" I asked, my fears for him dissipating. Dressed neatly, clean-shaven, and hair newly trimmed, his good humor was palpable.

He was carrying a small package that he placed on my desk. "I met a girl."

"Wonderful!" And somewhat surprising. I had expected him to do well academically but not necessarily socially. Still, security in one phase of life often means security in others. This is obviously what had happened inside Patrick.

"Tell me about her," I said.

"Her name is Sara." He grinned. "She's a nerd like me."

"You met her at school?"

"Yeah. She may not be beautiful to look at—though she's no dog, mind you—but her brain is beautiful. *She's* beautiful."

"She's interested in astronomy?"

"Of course. Otherwise she wouldn't be taking the course. She's twenty-seven, works in an architectural firm where she's going nowhere, and decided to change her life. Coincidence, isn't it?"

Or destiny, I thought. If Patrick hadn't decided to change his life, too, Sara and he almost certainly would never have met. I delighted in his joy.

"We're engaged," he said. "We'll marry in the winter. That's why I needed to see you, to tell you it wouldn't have happened without your help, to thank you in person."

"That's what therapy is for. I'm glad it worked so well."

He indicated the package he had put on my desk. "I brought you a present." I picked it up.

"Don't open it until I leave," he said, suddenly shy. "I hope you like it."

His mission fulfilled, he was obviously anxious to go, and I did not detain him. We shook hands, knowing we might never see each other again.

When he was gone, I opened the package. It was a book: H. G. Wells's *The Time Machine*.

CHAPTER 10

John:
Free Will and Destiny

I TALKED ABOUT FREE WILL and destiny earlier, and it forms a major theme in my previous book, *Only Love Is Real*. Yet it is a lesson that cannot be stressed enough, for it comes up frequently in our lives. Every day I hear about it from patients and from colleagues doing similar work.

Destiny and free will seem to exist together. There is an intelligence, a wisdom, or a consciousness that knows how events and relationships will turn out. Hamlet calls it a destiny "that shapes our ends." We on Earth don't know how they will end, but *we can affect how they will turn out for us both later in our life and in our lives to come by our present actions and behaviors—by our free will.*

Just as the soul does a review at the end of a life, so it seems to make a life preview before we are born. It plans the life. I'm going to work on compassion or empathy or nonviolence, for example. It sees how the life is set up, whom we're going to meet, who will help us along the spiritual path, and how we're going to help them. (It's complicated because there is an interaction with other souls, and they have their plans, too.) The people we meet and the experiences that are set up help us learn—this is destiny.

Okay. You've met this beautiful person, and you had in your life preview planned to spend the rest of your lives together, learning together, helping each other as you progress toward immortality. But the person is of the wrong religion or lives too far away, or your parents intervene, or you don't have the courage to override the influence of your culture, so you choose not to marry that person either spiritually or physically. This is free will. You had a choice and, freely made, it was no. The choice will bring you to a destiny point that might not have occurred if your choice had been yes. That is how we change our future in this life.

If you meet this person and marry, it will put you on one road that you chose with your free will, and it will affect the rest of this life and your future lives. If you choose to separate, you'll be on a different road, and you may be learning different lessons. You may meet a different soul mate or have a different experience. You will work primarily on empathy, say, rather than nonviolence. The more important questions are how quickly you are going to learn and how much happiness, spirituality, tranquility, and so forth, you are going to have in your life.

The answers depend to a large extent on your free will.

It is like climbing a tree: There are many different branches and many different choices. You'll come to the top of the tree eventually, but it may take five lifetimes or ten or thirty. How many lifetimes will it take to fulfill your soul's goal of learning compassion, for example? It will depend on the choices you make. Thus, both destiny (the tree, after all, was *there*) and free will coexist.

I don't believe in psychics who say, "You're going to meet this wonderful person in 2008, and you will be married." They may be skillful and talented psychics, and they may be right that you'll meet your partner in 2008, but it's free choice that will determine whether or not you spend your lives together. You'll choose based on your own intuition, not on the psychic.

* * *

Here is an example of a free choice made in the present that will change a man's future lives. It wasn't come by easily. Choices he made in earlier lives affected this one, and if he hadn't been able to regress and to understand the regression, I'm not sure how long it would have taken him to find the right path.

His name was John, and he died in what might have been the Great Fire of London. He wasn't sure of the date, only that it was a fire, it was in the Middle Ages, the city was London, and he died. The event traumatized him in the lifetimes to come.

I didn't know about it immediately. As with all my patients, we spent the first sessions discussing his present problems and trying to see if there was a root cause for them in his childhood or in other aspects of this current life. Then there were several regressions leading to dim and inconclusive images, and one that led to a vivid past but not to the fire.

The first thing I should know about him, he said almost as soon as we shook hands, was that he was rich. Usually, people tell you their age, where they live, their marital status, a little about their family history, or what they do for a living. Not John. "I'm a wealthy man," he said and then kept quiet as though that was all the information I needed.

I was tempted to say, "Well, good for you." Wealth doesn't impress me, and to boast about it seems not only bad manners but bad taste. But I quickly realized he wasn't boasting, for the statement was delivered without joy or pride. It was as though wealth was the problem he had come to see me about.

We would get to that. First, I wanted to study what he looked like and then take a conventional history.

Actually, John's appearance announced his wealth almost as directly as he did himself. He was in his early sixties and had the kind of mannequin looks that come with face-lifts, custom-made shirts, frequent Caribbean vacations (or a good sun lamp), teeth whiteners, a personal trainer, $200 haircuts, and a weekly manicure. I had the feeling that if someone struck him gently with a hammer, he would crumble like a new jerry-built facade on a rotting house. It wouldn't have surprised me if he had been or still was a professional model, though that did not seem a likely profession for him. Indeed, as it turned out, he had no profession at all.

He lived in a Palm Beach mansion with twenty rooms, servants, and a four-car garage. His wife, Lauren, was someone whose picture my wife, Carole, had seen not only in the society pages of the *Miami Herald* but also in articles about Florida society in *Vogue* and *Vanity Fair*. There was another house in Barbados, a flat in London, and a pied-à-terre in New York. There were also two children, Stacey, nineteen, in her sophomore year at Wellesley, "majoring in boys," John said, and Ralph, twenty-five, finishing law school and hoping to clerk for a Supreme Court justice. John was not optimistic about the boy's chances.

"What about you?" I asked. "Are your parents alive?"

"Died eight and ten years back."

"You had a good relationship with them?"

"I suppose so. They were very social. When I was a kid, I was brought up by nannies, but Mom and Dad often took me on trips with them. From the time I was twelve they sometimes let me have dinner with them when they had invited guests. When it was just the three of us, we ate together, of course, but that didn't happen often."

"Who were the guests likely to be?"

"Their friends, naturally—mainly the neighbors. When they came to dinner, I'd be there, too. They liked to play bridge after dinner, but by then I'd be in bed. And there were the business guests. My presence at such dinners was strictly verboten. Dad was what is called an 'international financier,' whatever that means. All sorts of illustrious bankers showed up, along with an occasional deposed dictator of some South American country and from time to time a European muck-a-muck. Margaret Thatcher slept over once. Quite a to-do."

"I'll bet. But not so good for a little boy."

"Not good at all," John said. "I always felt I was less important to my father than his business associates."

"And to your mother?"

"Less important than my father."

This was said as a kind of joke, but I could feel the pain beneath it. His mother had centered her attention on his father, not
on him. "Any siblings?"

"I'm an only child. They didn't have time to neglect more
than one."

"What about childhood friends?"

"Dozens of acquaintances, no close friends. My parents
would throw huge birthday parties for me, and it seemed every
child in Florida showed up, but I quickly realized they were there
for the food, the favors, and the pony rides, not because I was
close to their hearts. Even my school chums were only that—
chums. They were all nannied, too—closely supervised—so we
didn't have a chance to get into mischief. Even now I get jealous
when I hear about street gangs or reformatories. It seems to me
those boys had it better than I did."

His small ironies covered large wounds, I thought. It's hard to
be an adjunct to one's parents' lives. I knew from notes my assis-
tant jotted down when John first called for an appointment that
he had never sought psychotherapy before even though his unhappiness was long-standing, and I wondered what specific incident had impelled him to come to me.

"So you grew up overly cloistered?" I asked.

"Perfectly put. I was like a tapestry on their walls, beautiful
and finely crafted, but nothing more than an adornment." He
thought for a moment. "Still, I believe they loved me in their own
way."

"What about college? Surely you could escape then."

"All the way to the University of Southern California."

"And your life changed?"

"For the three months I was there."

"You were expelled?"

"Alas, nothing so dramatic. I quit."

"Why?"

"Because the work was too hard."

"You hated to study?"

"I *couldn't* study. There was no point in it. So it was too hard to pick up a book or a test tube."

"Isn't one point to get a degree?"

"I suppose so. I didn't need one to not work."

"Which even at eighteen you had mapped out as your future course?"

"Consciously, no, but subconsciously, yes."

"What about learning for the joy of it? For the intellectual excitement?"

"When I learn something, I feel no joy or excitement."

I was becoming exasperated. *"Nothing* interests you?"

"Many things do, but never for as long as a month. After I quit college, I tried a whole series of jobs: real estate, banking, Porsche salesman, sporting goods. None of them came to anything."

"How did your parents feel about that?"

"I'm not sure they knew. They certainly didn't care. You see, by the time I was twenty-one, my trust fund kicked in. One mil per year, enough for me to scrape by. I rented a house in Malibu and devoted myself to my one abiding interest: my since-I-was-fifteen obsession."

"Which is?"

"Girls. Women. The female form, the female flesh." He smiled. "As I say, from age fifteen, an obsession."

"So you had affairs, romances—"

"Absolutely. And one-night stands, fleeting dalliances. You name it. I never paid for sex, at least in the sense of hiring prostitutes or call girls, but my girls were expensive nevertheless. The finest dinners, a bauble or geegaw for the fabulous ones—at the very least a limousine ride home."

"How many were there?"

"Hundreds."

"And how long did the serious affairs last?"

"My usual concentration span: less than a month."

"But your wife—"

"Lauren. She was, of course, one of the fabulous ones, or else I wouldn't have married her."

"You've been married how long?"

"Twenty-six years."

"Sounds as if you've exceeded your concentration span by quite a lot."

"Not really. We've been married for a long time, true, but both of us lost interest quickly. With us it is more of a business arrangement."

My mind shuddered. "To lure—"

"Never! What do you take me for? No. Lauren's and my business is being rich. With our combined resources we can buy anything we want. *Anything*."

"Give me an example."

"Well . . . Madagascar."

"You bought Madagascar?"

He laughed. "Not really. Actually, our money goes toward good works. My parents funded a foundation for charitable work. It established start-up home tutoring programs for inner-city four- and five-year-olds from troubled families, set up AIDS clinics in seventeen different locations, with more to come—that sort of thing. And Lauren and I contribute heavily to it. The interest on the interest."

"But you don't take an active part in managing it?"

Another laugh, this time tinged with bitterness. "I couldn't manage a lemonade stand."

"Well, working for it, then. Looking for new projects."

He shrugged. "Too much work. Too much trouble."

"Does Lauren feel the same way?"

"She has her own public relations firm. It occupies her full-time, though God knows she doesn't need the income."

I decided to provoke him. His airy dismissal of any ambition, any goal, seemed a symptom of an unquiet soul. "While you stay home, doing whatever pleases you, working out but taking the occasional nap if it all gets too tough."

He glanced at me, stung. "Right in all but one respect: the occasional nap."

"Then ten hours of sleep each night is enough?"

The veneer cracked. His body sagged, and his eyes looked haunted. "Lately I haven't been able to sleep. Never on my own, and there isn't a drug powerful enough to keep me under for more than an hour or two."

"Yet you lead an ideal life: plenty of money, good looks, your pick of women, an understanding wife, a gorgeous home. Yes, you might have had neglectful parents, but they provided for you, and you tell me they loved you. What force is so powerful that it doesn't let you sleep?"

He struggled to keep his voice calm—and failed. "Terror, Dr. Weiss. Unremitting, abject terror."

I felt the hair rise on my arms. "Terror of what?"

"Of death. I run and run and run from the fear, but it always catches up. The women—they're just a diversion. So was any job I ever took. Nothing drove away the fear. It's hard to go outdoors—it was hard to come here—because I'm sure I'll be in an accident. I won't drive, can't drive. Our house has more alarm systems than a Mafia don's. We rarely travel; planes are death-traps. A sudden loud noise? I'm under the table. I'm a Vietnam vet with PTSD [post-traumatic stress disorder], only I've never been to war. The idea of my handling a gun is ludicrous. Jesus, I'm scared to carve a *turkey!* Last week I heard a car backfire, and I fainted, passed out. I decided it was crazy, and I'd better do something about it, so I called you."

He sat back, pale and shaken. I often find it difficult to figure out whether the causes of a patient's symptoms lie in his present life or some past-life event. Here, given John's present-life history, there seemed no question: Only something that had happened in a past life or a series of past lives could explain his trauma. I discussed the issue with him.

"I'm game," he said. "Nothing could be worse than what I'm already experiencing."

Our first attempts were inconclusive. It was as though John was reluctant to investigate the past. Eventually he reached a significant period, and it galvanized him.

"It's many centuries ago," John said, his eyes closed but his body tense. "I am a great warrior, a warrior-king. The army I lead is encamped outside a fortified city, its walls unbreachable because many of my men have grown sick from dysentery, and too few of them are well enough to mount an attack. Nevertheless, if we don't take the city, our weakness will become known, and we'll be slaughtered in the field. I've arranged a meeting with the ruler of the city, but before it takes place, I have my men pitch their tents and put on their armor to disguise the extent of our plight. What he sees before him when he looks at us from the battlements, I tell the ruler, is just a small portion of my army. Not five miles away is a force of three thousand men, only awaiting my signal before they attack. They have been without women for several months; the rape of his people's wives and daughters is only one of the consequences he can be sure of if the city falls. The men will be killed and the babies roasted on spits.

"My men have committed such atrocities in other battles, and word of them has reached the ruler, so he believes what I say. What will you have me do? he asks. Give up peacefully. Let us occupy your city only for the time it will take us to rest and care for our horses. Then we will leave. There are more important battles to be won elsewhere.

"The ruler agrees. He opens the gates to the city. Immediately my men attack. They kill all the able-bodied men. They ravish the women, and I rape the ruler's daughter, for I, too, have been too long without a woman's comfort. When we are finished, we set fire to the city, bolting the gates closed behind us as we depart. The fire spreads to the nearby woods, but my men are unharmed. All those within the city are burned to death. My name becomes synonymous with cruelty and destruction. I'm feared throughout the region. Great rulers give me untold riches to prevent my attacks. I can buy anything I want, have anything I want."

I led him back to the present. "Including Madagascar?" I asked when in his review he discussed his feeling of wealth and power.

He saw the connection between that past life and this present one, but my little joke didn't amuse him. He was staggered by the extent of his cruelty, horrified that in whatever life, in whatever persona, he was capable of rape and murder.

"I suspect you've paid for it," I said.

"In another life?"

"Precisely. In that life you remained unscathed. You must have been afraid somebody would take revenge on you"—he nodded—"but nobody did. The fear that you felt when you looked over your shoulder isn't commensurate with the terror you experience today."

He took a deep breath and exhaled with a sigh. "Then let's go back again."

It was to the time of the Great Fire. John was a wealthy merchant who neglected his wife and their two children in favor of countless affairs. His wife had left him, preferring to go penniless rather than stay with him, and she had taken the children with her. One of them, their six-year-old daughter, Alice, was visiting him, begging for money, when the fire broke out. He had fallen into a drunken sleep on his bed. His frantic daughter had been unable to rouse him when she first smelled the flames. It wouldn't have done either of them any good if she had. The fire was all-consuming, eating the wooden houses of London and everything else, alive or inanimate, they contained, and making the cobblestones so hot that escape was impossible.

"My first sensation was that I couldn't breathe," John said, gasping even as he relived it. "The smoke was so thick, it was impossible to see. I could hear Alice screaming as her hair caught fire, but the screams soon stopped. I supposed that, mercifully, she had died. Death came for me, too, but it took its time. The flames seemed to crawl their way up my body rather than taking me whole. My legs burned first, then my torso, and only after a long time my head. It was as though I was being crucified for sins like drunkenness and adultery—bad sins, I admit, but I didn't seem to deserve such a cruel sentence of death."

In his life review John realized that he *had* committed sins requiring the harshest punishment, only they were from his earlier life. He understood, too, why his fear was so great. There could be nothing worse than the agony he had experienced in London, and even the thought that it might happen again was unbearable. Rather than traumatizing him further, the visions of his cruelty and subsequent punishment by fire ignited in him impulses of compassion and charity. He took a far greater interest in his parents' foundation, at last channeling his great wealth into projects he oversaw himself; fittingly, one was the funding of auxiliary fire departments. He stopped womanizing, tried to heal the rift with Lauren (unfinished work that continues as I write this), and took courses in economics and management, expecting one day to take over the running of the foundation. He could sleep now, and with it came an energy that surprised him more than it did me. Compassion is energizing.

I continued to see him for many months, not to regress him but to discuss a lingering depression. He told me that no matter how much he devoted himself to acts of goodness, he couldn't do enough. I was able to assure him that he was on the right path and that there would be other lifetimes when he could put what he had learned more fully into practice.

Near the end of John's therapy sessions, he agreed to have me progress him into the near and distant future. Because of the benefits of his earlier regressions, he welcomed the idea of going forward. He had become an excellent hypnotic subject and had experienced vivid past life scenes. Perhaps he could do the same in the future.

Before John arrived for his progression, I thought about the power of destiny and free will. In the distant past, destiny had made him a leader of men; his sway over allies and enemies alike was enormous. Yet he had chosen to use his power and wealth for self-aggrandizement, for the subjugation of others, for the benefit of the few rather than the many. That decision had cost him in the lives that followed, both in London and in twenty-first-century Florida. If he had chosen another path—used his position for the benefit of his community and displayed compassion and love—then he would have had a different series of lives and would never have had to show up in my office, miserable and afraid. Our free will sometimes leads us to evil, not good; to selfishness, not selflessness; to insularity, not compassion; to hate, not love. We must learn that free will is dangerous if incorrectly used.

John's ability to go deep under hypnosis convinced me that his reports of his journeys into the future would be accurate, made up of what he had actually experienced rather than what he fantasized or wanted the future to be. He had the ability to put aside his cognitive mind, his intellect, in order to experience the future directly, without distortion.

Once again reaching a deep trance level, John moved ahead in time while maintaining an out-of-body awareness. He was quickly approached by two wise spiritual beings who led him to a fork in the road that indicated the way to future lifetimes. He telepathically "heard" from the wise men that one of the divergent paths, the one on the left, was the route he would have taken if he had not chosen compassion, charity, and generosity in his current lifetime. The one on the right was his reward for choosing wisely.

I led him down the path on the left so he could see what fate he had avoided through his current actions.

"I'm on a footbridge," he said, "surrounded by fog. But when I reach the other side, I can see clearly. I'm a woman named Diana, an American. It's maybe a hundred, maybe two hundred years from now—no more than that—and I'm carrying my baby girl home from a laboratory. I'm unhappily married to a hover-craft pilot who has long since stopped loving me and takes his sexual satisfaction from other women. So the baby's not his. I've never been pregnant. The baby is the result of an advanced cloning procedure. She'll literally be a little me, though I hope her life turns out more happily than mine. Cloning was perfected because human fertility and birth rates have declined precipitously due to the chemical toxins in the food, water, and air. Most people choose the lab method, and I'm glad I did. At least it's not my husband's child.

"I haven't traveled much, but my husband has. He's been all over the world in his hovercraft, which can go faster than the speed of sound. When he was still speaking to me, he reported that farms and forests have disappeared, that 'technology accidents' have made many areas uninhabitable, and that people live in huge city-states that are often at war with each other, further polluting the globe."

Life as Diana described it was not so different from now. People still suffered from the same problems and maladies. Science and technology had advanced, as often for ill as for good, but human ambition and prejudices had not changed. The world was a more dangerous place. Synthetic foods had helped allay hunger, but pollution threatened fish and the water supply. I brought her ahead in her life, and she began to cry.

"I thought my daughter would be a joy to me, but she turned

out to be as cold and cruel as my husband. I lived to be more than
a hundred years old, yet each day was a burden, a time of sadness.
Death was a relief. I was as alone when I died as I was throughout
my life."

I led John back to the fork in the road. Still in a deep state, he
understood immediately that he had learned how his London
wife felt when he, the wealthy merchant, had neglected her. It was
exactly what he felt when he became Diana and her husband de-
serted her.

John knew, however, that Diana was a figure in a life he would
not follow. He had chosen the road on the right, and I led him
along it now.

"I'm the president of a prestigious university in what had
been America before all national boundaries disappeared. I'm
immensely rich, but I live simply with my wife and three children in a house on the campus. I use my money for scholar-
ships, attracting the most talented people in the arts and
sciences to the university. I love working with them; their young
minds are full of fresh and innovative ideas. Together, they and
I and the fine faculty that teaches them look for ways to create
unity among the people of the earth by encouraging an emphasis on the similarities and not the differences between them. I
am a renowned man, but that means nothing compared to the
joy I get from life."

John's visit to this future was short; he would enjoy it fully
when it was time for him to go there. I instructed him to go beyond these two paths to a more distant future. He grinned happily, still in his deep state. "Which place do you want me to go?"
he asked. "I can transport myself anywhere I wish. People don't
need bodies anymore, though they can have them if they feel like
it. It's fun for sports, say, and surely for sex. But we can go anywhere and be anyone by using visualization and thought. We
communicate through consciousness and also through light
auras."

His own pleasure delighted me. "From the way you describe

it, this must be in the very, very distant future," I said, "many thousands of years from now."

"No," he answered, "not so distant as you think, though I can't tell you the year. The earth is very lush and green." (Again, this mirrored many of the other reports I was hearing.) "I can't see many people, but this may be because most don't wish to have bodies; they're happy being consciousness and light. The world is a transcendentally peaceful place, with no hint of war, violence, misery, or grief. I've been able to scan the planet for negative emotions; none exist. There's no evidence of anger, hatred, or fear. Just peace."

He could have stayed for hours in the future he was experiencing in my office, but by my watch it was a morning at the beginning of the twenty-first century and there was another patient in my waiting room, so I had to bring him back. When he came for his next session, he told me that he didn't want to return to the far future. "It was too beautiful," he said. "I have to live in the present, and for now that's beautiful enough."

John knew he had learned valuable lessons over his lifetimes and that there were many still to be learned. He realized that the choices he had recently made would profoundly affect his futures but that in those futures he would have to make different, equally important choices to reach the glories he had visualized in his travels far ahead. "But my choices alone won't produce that future," he said. "It is the collective decisions of all humans that will get us there."

Perhaps so. And perhaps that time is, as John has seen, "not so distant as you think."

CHAPTER 11

Contemplation and Meditation

I AM DAILY making myself what I am." The quote comes from Robert Thurman, the eminent Buddhist scholar at Columbia University, and to me it is an energizing thought. I love the concept of process and flux that it implies.

Every day you are new. Your thoughts, your intentions and actions, your awareness and perceptions are constantly evolving, and with each shift a different you emerges. You are not the same person you were five years ago or even five minutes ago. And neither are your loved ones, your friends, or your acquaintances. One result is that often we react to the old person—and they react to us—as we once knew them, so that, for example, the high school bully remains a bully to us when we see him again even though he might have found spiritual peace and is the mildest mannered of men.

So evolution isn't much good if you aren't aware of it. How can you mature if you don't see the process at work? How can you learn from life if you don't stop to experience it? How can you embody all that has happened to you physically and psychologically if you don't give your body and mind the time to ingest it? How can you change as your friends and loved ones change?

The way to assess ourselves and others is through relaxed spiritual contemplation and meditation, and the time to start is in the present. There is a difference between them, although they are close kin. Contemplation means concentrating on a specific subject or object—the idea of loving kindness, for example, or the beauty of a butterfly. Meditation requires keeping the mind completely blank, in a state of mindfulness or awareness, free to accept whatever feelings, ideas, images, or visions enter it and letting associations flow to all aspects of the object or thought—to understand its form, shape, color, *essence*. It is the art of observing without thought, without mental comment. It is far easier for the Western mind to practice contemplation. We are used to focusing our brains on a given subject, thinking about it, and analyzing it. Meditation is more of an Eastern concept, difficult to grasp and requiring a great deal of practice. It takes months or years to be able to meditate whole-mindedly, and you might not be able to fully master it in this one lifetime. That doesn't mean, however, that you shouldn't try meditating now. (Remember: In this life, as in all others, you are consciously progressing toward immortality.) The attempt itself brings its own profound rewards, and you will soon find yourself looking forward to the time of aloneness that meditation requires.

You might want to start with contemplation, and the object to concentrate on is yourself. To find out who you are now, think of yourself in the moment. Let whatever thoughts you have about yourself, good and bad, enter your consciousness. Which negative or judgmental images and feelings would you discard as no longer accurate or valid? Which positive and self-healing impressions and feelings would you now add? What life experiences have shaped you most profoundly? When you have another life, what do you imagine would change from this one? The point is not to "like" yourself or, indeed, pass judgment of any kind. You are trying to see what is really there beneath the camouflage of the person you show to the world.

Consider the significant people in your life. Are your images of them outdated? Has your own experience taught you to look at them differently? How have they changed as you yourself have changed? How will these changes lead you to modify your relationship with them in a more positive, understanding, and loving manner? How will they facilitate further change?

We are all works in progress, moving at different speeds along our spiritual paths. But daily we should pause to involve the creative mind on the core concepts that can shape us as humans wishing to rise toward the One: love, joy, peace, and God.

Contemplation and meditation aren't easy, for the further inward you go, the more deeply felt will be your understanding, and going deep requires digging through layers of defenses. We are so disciplined to think and analyze that attempts to clear or empty the mind defy our training. Yet analysis is counter to contemplation and meditation, and we must shed it as we begin to explore. It isn't enough to say to yourself, "I'm ridding my mind of all things except the notion of loving kindness," or, going further, "I'm ridding my mind of all thoughts whatsoever and am aware of nothing and everything at once." In both cases you will find yourself distracted by the outside world. You might be able to think about loving kindness for a while, but I'll bet that soon you will remember a time when you weren't kind or someone wasn't kind to you, and from that might come the thought: "My God! It's Mother's birthday, and I forgot to call her" or some other notion that whisks you back to everyday matters. And if you try to blank your mind entirely, you'll almost surely find it filling with mundane distractions: your nose itches or there is a housefly in the room or the thought that if you keep sitting much longer, you'll miss the rerun of *Seinfeld*.

* * *

The present discussion is mostly about meditation, but much of what follows is applicable to contemplation as well.

Meditation stills the chatter that normally fills our minds, and the resulting quiet allows us to observe without judgment, to reach a higher level of detachment, and eventually to become aware of a higher state of consciousness.

A simple exercise can demonstrate how difficult it is to keep your mind devoid of thoughts, feelings, to-do lists, physical discomforts, everyday worries, or household or business concerns.

After reading this paragraph, close your eyes for a minute or two. (I suggest sitting in a favorite chair or on a comfortable cushion or in bed. Be as comfortable as possible.) Take a few deep breaths, exhaling away all the stresses and tensions you carry around in your body. Try to keep your mind calm and think of nothing, not even beautiful sunsets or gentle seas. The object is to still your left brain, the part that thinks and analyzes. Ready? Begin now.

It didn't work, did it?

You probably had several moments of relaxation and pleasure, but then you might have thought about how silly you looked holding an open book with your eyes closed. And then perhaps about a report: Would you make the deadline for it? Or did you forget the mint jelly for the leg of lamb you are serving your guests tonight? The stresses of today's world seem to intrude constantly into our daily lives, and in an artificial-seeming environment—in solitude in a darkened silent room—they seem to pummel us. Under this barrage of stress the physical body seems to function at a higher level of alertness—the so-called fight-or-flight reaction—triggering a host of psychological reactions. You might even feel fear, thinking that the silence is somehow threatening. (Many of us turn on the radio or television as soon as we get home, often to ward off the dread of the assault of thoughts or memories.) So how long have you been sitting still? Five minutes? It seems a good start, you tell yourself, though you know it isn't. Perhaps you'll be able to give yourself another minute or so tomorrow, as though meditation was something to endure.

Maybe, you tell yourself the next day, rather than meditate you'll contemplate. Not yourself—it is too dangerous to begin there—but, as Dr. Weiss suggests, you'll concentrate on loving kindness. Contemplation, you have read, will engage your mind, leading you to a deeper understanding of kindness in today's session, since that is its subject, and eventually leading to yourself and the life around you. And understanding leads to freedom, joy, self-fulfillment, and better relationships: that is, happiness.

To contemplate a thought or concept is to focus on its meaning, and, as noted, it is easier than emptying the mind and observing, the essence of meditation. As you focus, different levels of meaning will emerge. Also, your mental associations with the core object or concept will lead you down further avenues of insight and understanding. It is okay to think during contemplation as long as you keep your focus.

What images does the term *loving kindness* conjure up? Perhaps a person (your mother? grandmother?) or some act you did spontaneously or some act you were the recipient of? Maybe a *feeling*, a warmth that pervades your body and brings forth a tear of happiness? Once you have located the image or feeling, you'll come to an understanding of the more general definition of the phrase. Loving kindness is a spiritual act, and to focus on the spiritual can be extremely rewarding.

Your entire value system will change for the better if loving kindness resides at the base of it. You will find that fears and anxieties are reduced or even eliminated. Your thought process will lead you from your basic definition to a clearer understanding of your spiritual nature. (You see, you are contemplating yourself after all!) In time, with the awareness of what that spiritual essence is, a sense of inner peace, patience, balance, and harmony will manifest itself in your daily life.

Physical benefits also accrue. With the diminution of fear and anxiety and the arrival of inner tranquility, the body is strengthened. The immune system is enhanced. I have seen chronic illnesses alleviated in the bodies of patients whose minds are at peace. Some people have noted energy shifts when insights and understandings emerge. The mind and body are so intimately connected that healing one heals the other.

Sometimes when you focus on a concept, you may discover that what comes up differs from what your training, education, or history has taught you. This is to be expected since we have all been indoctrinated with the belief systems and values of our families, teachers, cultures, and religions. That you now see things in a new way will not hurt you. Keeping an open mind is essential. If you can attune your mind to different ideas and new possibilities, then the learning process can continue.

Perhaps what you were taught as a baby or child is not what you are experiencing now. How can you know unless your mind is active and aware? How can you awaken to a deeper or more meaningful reality unless you allow your mind to function in an open manner, making no judgments until you have mentally tested every option for yourself? Try not to dismiss or discard ideas or brush aside what you experience because they are different from what you were led to believe. It is possible that the strange might be true, the familiar false.

When you contemplate, take your time. By definition, contemplation implies an unhurried mental focus. Your mind must reflect on its responses and perhaps add another reflection and response to the first—and then another and another. You may find memories popping into your awareness like stars in the early evening sky. You may experience sudden clarifying insights with their attendant healing effects.

I recommend contemplating one thing at a time, to ensure that you provide the proper depth and duration to your experience. Even then it is unlikely that one session will bring you to the core of the object or concept being contemplated. You can and should return to the object or concept until you master it, fully understand it, and are aware of the changes within you that it has wrought. It is then that you will be amazed and delighted at the beauty and power of your insights, liberated by the healing effects of your understanding.

When you believe you have found the core, don't stop your contemplation. Begin a new contemplation on the same concept the following day. Close your eyes and take a few relaxing breaths. Imagine you can actually exhale the tensions and stresses in your body and that you are inhaling pure, healing energy. Relax your muscles and let the core of the concept or object reappear in your awareness. For approximately the next ten minutes consider all the levels of meaning that this thought or object holds for you. Loving kindness is a profound spiritual concept, but there is profundity, too, in a butterfly's beauty. Consider the implications. How will your life change with new understanding? Your relationships? Your values? Take your time. There is no hurry and no test at the end. Savor your insights and instructions. Remind yourself that you'll remember everything you are experiencing.

If your mind wanders and you lose focus, don't criticize yourself. It is normal for your thoughts to drift away, and all you need to do is gently return to the subject. After some practicing, you will notice that even when your mind strays, there is still a connection to the original thought; in psychiatry we call this free association. The more you practice, the easier it is to maintain focus and the deeper and more profound your understandings are. So try to let any frustrations float away, but don't compel yourself to sit and contemplate if the outside world is too much with you. Try again tomorrow. Pleasure is a vital component to contemplation and meditation. The purpose is to become free, not to chain yourself to the process.

After you have finished and your eyes have opened and your mind has returned to everyday consciousness, you might want to record your experience in a journal or on tape. This is a way to solidify your thoughts and aid your memory for future insights.

Many people find it fascinating to return to the concept weeks or months after they have "mastered" it and to compare this journey with the previous one. There are no rules in this regard. Trust your intuitive wisdom. As the Christian mystic Pierre Teilhard de Chardin said, "You are not a human being having a spiritual experience; you are a spiritual being having a human experience." There is meaning in everything, and purity of spirit when you find it.

As rewarding as contemplation is, meditation is still the means for going as deeply into the spiritual realm as is humanly possible. Here you are not bound by a single concept or confined by concentration. Rather, you are saying to your mind, body, and soul, "You are free to go wherever you want in your search for spiritual progression. You are not constrained by time or place but can travel to the past or to the future, to lands known or unknown, to places as small as the human heart or as vast as the universe."

Believe me, there is no more inspiring journey.

I have written a book entirely on meditation *(Meditation: Achieving Inner Peace and Tranquility in Your Life)*, yet I have not come close to achieving the wisdom and spiritual peace described by the yogis and monks of Asia who have spent their entire lives devoted to it. For me and for you the point is not to reach meditative "perfection" but to get as much out of the practice as we can, to use it as one of many tools in our evolution, to point us toward spirituality, and to help us therapeutically.

Before I met Catherine, my medical education had followed orthodox lines and my psychiatric training had been by-the-book traditional. But after my experience with her, I began to explore alternative therapies; it was during this quest that I learned the value of meditation.

Like hypnosis, which I use as a tool to regress patients to their past lives, meditation develops the ability to open the mind to the deepest, most hidden influences on our bodies and souls, whether they come from past, future, or present lives. Paradoxically, by thinking of nothing, by clearing the mind, we are free to *remember*. The memories of past, present, and future lives help us locate the origins of our traumas, and once they are revealed to us, we can recognize that our fears come from another place and are no longer a threat. I have had memories of my own past lives during deep meditation and have thereby gained insights into my behavior, my defenses, and my fears. I would not be as self-knowing as I am today (and there is lots more to learn) if I had not meditated.

We can also use meditation to resolve personal conflicts and difficult relationships or to help the heart to heal. But eventually for all of us the primary purpose of meditation is to achieve inner peace and balance through spirituality.

Monks can meditate for hours. You should start with twenty minutes. Sit comfortably or lie down if you wish, though there is the possibility of falling asleep. Close your eyes; breathe slowly, regularly, and deeply; locate any areas of tension in your body (with me it is the neck and shoulders); and send your body a message: *Everything is fine. Everything is at peace. Relax.*

Let scattered thoughts and everyday concerns float gently out of your mind. Block out the clamoring voices of work, family, obligation, and responsibility that usually assail you—one by one if necessary. Mentally watch them vanish. Live *this* moment, this precious, unique moment of grace, light, and freedom, by surrendering to it.

Because the present is the only place you can find happiness, joy, peace, and freedom, psychospiritual practice emphasizes mindfulness of the present moment such as I have just described. The human mind is a creative masterpiece; by giving it rein, it can transport us to the heights of joy. Mindfulness is the awareness of those thoughts, emotions, feelings, and perceptions that are occupying us now and only now. By eliminating the distraction of the immediate past and worries about the future, the act of meditating opens the door to inner peace and health.

By carrying us from everyday awareness into the mindfulness of the present moment—*only* this moment, this precise instant—and thus into the spiritual values that elevate our souls, meditation frees us to go anywhere. Along the way we may gain clarity about a present trauma, a past or future life, or an unconscious denial of the nature of our problems. That is meditation's therapeutic value; the unaware becomes aware. But it may simply illuminate the reality of the beauty of the moment and all the wonder it contains. This is what is called *insight,* and it is how we come to ultimate reality.

Here is an illustration of mindfulness:

I was teaching a patient of mine, Linda, how to meditate. One day she came to me in great excitement. "I just saw the most beautiful tree!" she said.

"Where?" I asked, intrigued.

"Why, in front of my house."

Meditation had opened Linda's eyes to the beauty that had been within her reach all the time, only she had neglected to see it. Linda, a grade school teacher, was habitually rushing because she was late to her classes, but meditation had taught her to slow down.

Stephan Rechtschaffen, the director of the Omega Institute in Rhinebeck, New York, tells of the time when he was in his office discussing a business problem with a colleague. It was a beautiful spring day, and from his window he could see a guest at the institute, the Vietnamese Buddhist monk and philosopher Thich

Nhat Hanh, walking across the lawn. "With each step, he was kissing the earth. He was totally present, obviously immersed only in the act of walking. I could almost *feel* him savoring each moment, feel the sensation of grass on sole, feel the way his body seemed at one with each movement." *

Thich Nhat Hanh was living in the moment, just as Linda had learned to do. "In us," the monk writes, "there is a river of feelings, in which every drop of water is a different feeling, and each feeling relies on all the others for its existence. To observe it, we just sit on the bank of the river and identify each feeling as it surfaces, flows by, and disappears." *

When we meditate, we are sitting on that riverbank.

In *Meditation: Achieving Inner Peace and Tranquility in Your Life,* I share a message that came to me in a meditation which might be similar to one of your own:

> With love and understanding comes the perspective of infinite patience. What's your hurry? There *is* no time, anyway; it only feels that way to you. When you're not experiencing the present, when you're absorbed in the past or worried about the future, you bring great heartache and grief to yourself. Time is an illusion, too. Even in the three-dimensional world, the future is only a system of probabilities. Why do you worry so?
>
> The past must be remembered and then forgotten. *Let it go.* This is true for childhood and past-life traumas; but it's also true for attitudes, misconceptions, and belief systems that have been drummed into you, and for all old thoughts—indeed, for *all* thoughts. How can you see freshly and clearly with those thoughts?

* From *Time Shifting,* Doubleday, 1996.

What if you needed to learn something new, and with a fresh perspective?

Stop thinking. Instead, use your intuitive wisdom to experience love again. Meditate. See that everything is interconnected. See your true self. See God.

Meditation and visualization will help you to stop thinking so much and will help you begin the journey back. Healing will occur. You will begin to use your unused mind. You will see. You will understand. And you will grow wise. Then there will be peace.

The only thing I'd add now is what I've learned since the passage was written: You will not only begin the journey back, but you will begin the journey into the future.

Meditation can help us tap into the healing powers within us, not only psychic healing but physical healing as well. More and more, physicians are acknowledging that we can fight diseases, even very serious ones, with a recently discovered medicine: the curative powers that lie within our spiritual nature. (Recently discovered in the West, that is; Eastern doctors have known about it for centuries.) Perhaps this is true holistic medicine where we energize the entire organism—the mind and spirit as well as the body.

There is by now ample proof. In *Head First: The Biology of Hope and the Healing Power of the Human Spirit* (Dutton, 1989), Norman Cousins detailed how emotions affect the immune system; researchers at Harvard have found that meditation can prolong life in the elderly; and doctors in England found that diet, exercise, and the practice of stress-reduction techniques, of which meditation is among the most important, can actually *reverse* coronary artery disease. Diet and exercise alone won't do it.

The power of prayer on healing has also been documented— not only one's own prayers and prayers by family and friends but the prayers of strangers. In 1982, for instance, 393 patients in the coronary care unit of San Francisco General Hospital were randomly selected to either receive or not receive intercessory prayers. Neither the patients nor the doctors and nurses knew which group was which. The patients who received prayers had less need of CPR, mechanical ventilators, diuretics, and antibiotics, and there were fewer instances of pulmonary edema and even fewer deaths. In a study conducted by Duke University and the Durham Veteran Affairs Medical Center, heart patients who were prayed for by seven different religion groups from various places of the globe had better outcomes than those receiving traditional medical treatment alone. A study of patients with advanced AIDS found that when people prayed for them from afar, without the AIDS victims even knowing they were being prayed for, they experienced fewer and less severe AIDS-related illnesses, fewer and shorter hospitalizations, and less depression.

I teach my patients meditation techniques that can reduce insomnia, help with weight control, smoking cessation, stress reduction, fighting infections, and chronic illness, and lowering blood pressure. The techniques work because the chemistry and physics of the body are influenced by mental and physical energies; regular meditation is a priceless tool for the recovery and maintenance of health.

Meditation can open up possibilities for spiritual experiences since the subconscious mind is one of the gateways to the eternal dimension. The gateway is never wide open, and there are no signs that advise us where the road will lead. No code or magic word will open it; it is an interior process of transforming and being transformed. Put differently, the mind is a passage, and through meditation you will in time be possessed of a map by which you will be able to find your way along that passage into deeper, more transcendent states.

Meditation might bring you to a heightened awareness of your spiritual essence and to a state of profound ecstasy, lightness, satisfaction, and well-being that comes when we contact our deepest dimension. Meditation allows a feeling of bliss to spread through you when you are contemplating a concept or object that gives you pleasure. It may bring you back to a past life or ahead to a future one; the lessons of each will be clear to you when you enter them.

When you come to awareness, you will find yourself compassionate and loving without expecting anything in return. You will feel a oneness with every other person and being, with nature, with the sky and sea—with all there is. For however long you are in this altered state, you will experience the ultimate "high," a feeling unique in each individual yet common to the souls who are further along on their evolutionary journey. Some of my patients have told me that during meditation they detach from their physical bodies and float above themselves, watching themselves from another realm, the same out-of-body experience reported by people who have returned from near death. You may share that experience or have adventures as yet unreported by anyone. One thing is certain: You will discover your most powerful and essential self.

CHAPTER 12

David:
Spirituality

W HEN I WAS A YOUNG BOY, I would go to temple with my
father on Saturday morning and watch the old men
sway and rock *(daven)* as they recited their prayers. These were
always the same prayers, my father told me, said throughout
the day, morning, sundown, and night. I didn't understand the
language of the prayers, Hebrew, but, more fundamentally,
I couldn't understand the reason for them. "It doesn't make
sense," I thought. "The words can't continue to have meaning
after so many years, and by this time the swaying and bowing
can't be more than physical exercise."

After Catherine, I understood. The men were putting themselves in an altered state, just as I put patients under hypnosis. I
don't think it mattered what the content of the words was; it was
the ritual that mattered. The men were making a connection with
God, and the ritual—as with all religious rituals, no matter what
the religion—enabled them to become more spiritual. Whether
one is Jewish, Christian, Islamic, the object is the same: to come
closer to the supreme spiritual being and, by doing so, to become
closer to pure spirituality itself.

To me being spiritual means to be more compassionate, car-

SAME SOUL, MANY BODIES ———— 181

ing, and kind. It means reaching out to people with a loving heart without expecting anything in return. It means acknowledging something greater than one's self, a force that exists in an unknown realm that we must strive to discover. It means understanding that there are higher lessons to be learned and, after we have learned them, knowing that there are higher lessons still. The capacity for spirituality is in each of us, and we must tap into it.

I've seen religious people committing acts of violence and inciting others to acts of war. Kill, they say, for those you attack do not share our beliefs and thus are our enemies. These people haven't learned the lesson that there is but one universe, one soul. To me their attitude is completely *un*spiritual, no matter what the religion espouses. Indeed, it marks the difference between religion and spirituality. You do not need religion to be spiritual; you can be an atheist and still be kind and compassionate. You can do volunteer work, for example, not because God commands you but because doing it makes you feel good and you think this is the way human beings should act toward one another, that this is the way to progress toward the higher realm.

My conception of God is of a loving, wise energy that is in every cell of our bodies. I do not see him as the standard cliché of a man with a beard sitting on a cloud making judgments. (In psychoanalytical terms, this is projection, the anthropomorphizing of God.) The important question regarding spirituality is not which God you follow but are you true to your soul? Are you living a spiritual life? Are you a kind person here on earth, getting joy from your existence, causing no harm, and doing good to others?

This is the essence of life, essential to our journey upward, and it doesn't seem complicated. But too many of us haven't yet mastered these lessons of spirituality. We are selfish, materialistic, and lacking in empathy and compassion. Our urge to do good is subsumed by our desire to be physically comfortable.

And as goodness and selfishness battle within us, we become confused and unhappy.

That is the way it was with David, as you'll see.

David's family was patrician, from old New England stock, and he had come all the way from Boston to see me. He had heard of the work I was doing and had found one of my regression CDs helpful in relaxing him, though he had not experienced a past life. Besides, he had tried conventional psychotherapy, and it had done him little good.

"I have planned to stay a week," he said. "Can we accomplish anything in that time?"

"We can try," I replied, noting the impeccable cut of his trousers and the polo pony insignia on his shirt. "I can schedule you for three sessions. But we can't do anything until you tell me what brought you here."

To my surprise, the question seemed to puzzle him. "I'm not sure," he said at last. "I'm—I'm unhappy."

"Professionally? Personally?"

"Both . . . Neither."

"Which?"

"The point is I *shouldn't* be unhappy."

"Unhappiness isn't a matter of 'should.' It's a state of mind."

"Yes, of course. Only when I think about my life, which is far more frequently than I'd wish, I can't see a single thing to be unhappy about."

"Your profession?" I asked.

"Attorney. I work in my father's firm, and I've been doing well. Made partner in two years, and if I say so myself, it wasn't because of nepotism."

Still, there's often friction when a son works for a parent. "Do you find it uncomfortable being accountable to your father?"

"Not at all," he said emphatically, punctuating his words with a little clap of his hands. "My father lets me operate independently. He brought me up to be my own man, and so did my mother. He never second-guesses me and hardly ever sees me in the office. I think I spend more time with him socially than I do at work."

When psychiatrists begin the search for the root of a patient's problem, they often look at the family first. Was some unconscious dynamic at work here that David did not recognize?

I probed further. "Is your mother alive?"

"And kicking." He smiled. "She's on the board of the opera, the ballet, the Museum of Fine Arts. *And* she's a great hostess." He raised a hand, anticipating my question. "Yes, she had plenty of time for me when I was a kid, and plenty of time for my brother and sister, too. We have a great relationship."

"You said you see your father socially."

"And my mother, too, of course. Theirs has been a solid marriage for forty years."

"How often?"

"Maybe once a week. More like three times a month."

"You're married?"

Another hand clap. "Absolutely. To the divine Leslie."

Was he being ironic? "She's also a lawyer?"

"No, but she's in an allied profession. She's an actress. I met her in my second year at Harvard law. Went to a performance of *The Winter's Tale* at the Brattle Street Theatre and was so knocked out by her Perdita that I went backstage and asked her out. It's to my everlasting good fortune that she said yes then and yes when I asked her to marry me five years ago."

"Did your parents approve?"

" 'Boston scion weds lowly actress'? I don't know how they felt at first. As I said, they let me make my own life choices. But by now they adore her."

"Any children?"

"None. But that won't be true in another five months. Amniocentesis says it's a boy. *Voilà*. The line continues! The name carries on!"

He told me all this with a sense of pleasure, even of fun. Now he leaned forward, and his expression darkened. "Dr. Weiss, that's just the point. I love my parents, had a wonderful childhood, have a spectacular wife, am well educated, well fed, well clothed and housed. We have enough money to stave off any disaster or to take us anywhere on the planet we want to go. I am truly the man without a care in the world. Yet when I think these things, and even though I know they're true, there's a fundamental problem: The man I've just described isn't the man living inside my skin."

This last was accompanied by a sob and a look of anguish so intense that I actually thought I was facing a different man. "Can you be more specific?" I asked.

He recovered with an effort. "I wish I could be. When I try to put into words how I feel, it sounds like whining. The paltry complaints of an overprivileged narcissist."

"It doesn't matter how it sounds, and obviously the complaints aren't paltry. You're in pain."

He gave me a look of gratitude and took a deep breath. "Okay. Here goes: I don't know why I was put on this Earth. I feel as if I'm skating on a frozen pond called life and that underneath the water is a hundred feet deep. I know I should swim in it, that it'd be good if I could experience it, but I don't know how to break through the ice. I'm confused about my place in the world. Yes, I'm happy working for my father, but that's only one definition of me: my father's son. I'm more. And I'm more than another definition: good husband about to become good father. Jesus," he went on, the words startlingly loud in my office, "I'm bloody invisible. Life just whistles through me like wind."

His need for answers ran deep, I knew. Rather than whiney, his complaints were existential, a cry for a definition he had not been able to find.

Perhaps he had been looking in the wrong place.

* * *

David told me that when he used my CDs at home, he generally got so relaxed that he fell asleep. There is nothing wrong with that; it simply means the person is going too deep. But his earlier "practice" made the hypnotic induction in my office easier. Within minutes he was in a deep trance.

"It's the twelfth century," he said slowly, as though trying to peer into his life from the outside. "I'm a nun, Sister Eugenie, and I work at a hospital on the outskirts of Paris." He shuddered. "It's a dreadful place, dark and cold, and my life is very hard. All the beds are filled in the room where I work, and I know there are others outside waiting for someone to die so they can have the space. The patients' bodies are covered with blisters—blisters filled with fluid. The smell is awful. Even in the cold these poor people run high fevers. They sweat and groan. Their torment is terrible to see.

"I don't mind working there. One of the patients is an eleven-year-old girl, an orphan, eyes bright with fever, lips parched, face wrinkled like a monkey's. We both know she's going to die, that there's nothing I can do for her. Nevertheless, her spirits are good, she's able to make jokes, and the other patients love her. I love her most of all, and I bring her water and wash her brow—I do this for everyone—with a special tenderness.

"On the day she dies, she looks up at me and says, 'You came into my life and brought me peace. You made me happy.' *Happy!* Can you imagine that? This poor girl, in agony, says she's happy because of me. I'm not sure of the reason, but I redouble my efforts for the other patients, hoping I can bring the same happiness or at least some peace to them as well. And it works! I know my presence soothes them, and bonds form between us—spiritual bonds, though none as strong as between me and the orphan girl."

His face reflected his own inner peace as he spoke. His voice was gentle, awed, aware of miracles.

"Eventually, I, too, succumbed to the disease. The pain was excruciating, but though my body suffered, my mind and soul were blissful. I knew I had led a useful life, and that was God's plan for me.

"When I die, my soul flows upward, toward the God who had sustained me. I'm enveloped in a golden light and feel renewed by his grace. Angelic beings arrive to escort me, greeting me with applause and heavenly songs. On Earth I have risked my own life to help others with no thought of material gain. *This* was my reward, more valuable than a king's treasure, more precious than emeralds.

"They give me knowledge, and in exchange I give them boundless love. Through them I understand that helping others is the highest good, and you can imagine my joy when they tell me I had achieved that. The length of one's life is not important, they say. The number of days and years one lives on Earth is insignificant. It's the quality of those days and years that's important, quality measured in loving acts and achieved wisdom. 'Some people do more good in one day than others do in a hundred years.' This is their message. 'Every soul, every person is precious. Every person helped, every life aided or saved, is immeasurably valuable.'

"Each soul I attended in that hospital, belonging to those whose bodies had perished before mine, send me their blessings and their love, compounding my joy."

David paused. "An incredibly beautiful being differentiates itself from the chorus of angels," he continued. "It seems to be made of light, though it has a distinctively human form and wears purple robes and golden shoes. Its voice—not distinguishable as a man's or a woman's—has the authority of great wisdom."

When I led him back to the present, he was still under the power of his vision, still filled with awe and enlightenment. "Let's call that being the Source," he told me, "because it was obvious that the lessons the angels taught me were taught to them by it. 'When you need aid, you can invoke it through meditation and prayer whenever you need in any incarnation,' the Source instructed me directly. 'An open and loving heart, seeking a higher good without selfish motive, without any shadow of negativity or harm, can invoke a powerful manifesting energy in order to accomplish its goals. This is our right as spiritual entities. This is an essence of our spirituality. This is the invocation of grace.' "

He shook his head in wonder. "I've never had such thoughts in my life," he said. "I'm not religious. Don't believe in God and don't have the foggiest idea what part of me the Source came from. The idea that I was once a nun—it seems preposterous."

"It was a life you lived," I said. "Surely an important one, since you got to it so quickly and it was so vivid."

"It couldn't have been a fantasy," he agreed. "It's too remote from anything I've imagined in the past."

"So you think it's real?"

He held up a hand. "Whoa! I wouldn't go that far. But I'll tell you this, Dr. Weiss. It was the most amazingly moving experience I can remember."

"Maybe Sister Eugenie is the person inside your skin," I said. "Maybe she's the David you're looking for."

He thought for a moment. "We'll have to see, won't we?" The session was over. He stood and then clapped his hands. "What's next?"

When he came back two days later, he told me the past life had stayed in his mind from the moment he left, and he felt he had experienced a kind of epiphany. He was very curious now about the "next," and he virtually flung himself into the chair.

Within minutes he was transported back some 140 years to the American Civil War. This time he stayed outside his vision, although he saw it clearly. He was a young man on the Union side, an infantry soldier who spent his days either marching or fighting. "It's battle after battle," he said. "Each one worse than the last. I'm afraid to make friends because I'm sure they'll be killed or wounded. That's what happens to all of them: mutilated or killed. The men we're fighting, they're not our enemies, they're our brothers. The only reason we shoot at them is so they won't shoot us first. I try to save as many of my comrades as I can, help them find shelter or give them food or water. I do the same for our enemies when it's possible." He cast his eyes down as though trying not to see. "It's all so senseless and sad. It's impossible to tell victory from defeat. Brother killing brother interminably. Over what? An acre? A stream? An idea?"

He seemed suddenly sad and old. "I didn't survive the war, either. I just gave up and let myself be killed by walking into the battle from behind a tree. I didn't have the energy to fight or the stomach to kill anymore. It was a kind of assisted suicide." He sighed resignedly. "Wars, epidemics, earthquakes—all of nature's disasters or man's. Calamities that kill hundreds or hundreds of thousands—the cost is incalculable." His tone became confidential. "Some, which seem unavoidable, are really not. They can be mitigated by our own consciousness, by our collective thoughts and intentions. The others, which seem avoidable, only require the will to prevent them."

He was talking about saving lives by preventing violence, but did he mean that natural disasters could be prevented by the use of human will? I wasn't sure, and David, when he returned to the present, didn't know, either. Perhaps future regressions would help him explain.

Before he left on this day, David glimpsed some scenes of a past life in China many centuries ago (he could not pinpoint the year). As soon as he arrived in that life, his body began to shake, and I asked him if he wanted to come back.

"No," he said quickly. "I'm not frightened or sick. Besides, I'm just watching. I'm an eleven-year-old boy. My body is shaking because the ground is shaking. It's an earthquake. My family is rich, and they built the strongest house possible. But it can't stand against nature's force. The walls are crumbling. I hear the screams of my parents, of my brother and sister. Frantic, I race to help them, but it's too late. My little sister is barely alive, and I hold her in my arms until she dies. I run to another room. It does no good. The walls collapse, and I die with the rest of them."

Almost as soon as David entered that life, he left it. He had come simply for the lessons it offered him. "My life was short and happy," he observed when he was once again in the present. "Buildings were flimsy; they couldn't resist the tremors. In that time the devastation couldn't have been avoided, not with the level of knowledge or awareness then. But now we have the knowledge, and still people die. It's infuriating. We continue to build flimsy structures in dangerous areas with little planning and preparation. And I'm not talking about only Third World countries, I'm talking about America, too! It's not the lack of money that's stopping us but the lack of value placed on human life. We'd rather sacrifice people than spend money that we have. Simple safety measures could avoid pain, hurt, and even death. Each life is so important, so special, and yet thousands are sacrificed, usually for greed." Another sigh. "When will we learn?"

I had no answer, though I had been thinking the same thing for years. Perhaps when we are all as enlightened as David. Perhaps when we realize that when one person dies, it is part of our own process of dying. All lives and souls are connected.

When David came back for his final session, we visited two additional past lives. Again the theme in his previous regressions manifested itself, and he was able to articulate it: There is a supreme value in helping others because each life, each physical manifestation of the soul's journey, is absolutely precious.

In the first past life that day he was a doctor in the Roman Empire during what appeared to him to be an outbreak of the plague. He saw himself wrapping bandages around the legs of his patients, not because of their wounds but because the bandages would ward off fleas which, he deduced, came from infected rats and carried the hideous disease to humans. He warned everyone to stay away from all rats, particularly dead ones (the fleas would leave the corpses), and to keep themselves clean and indoors as much as possible. He saved many lives, but the epidemic raged on in the areas where his advice was not known or not followed. Miraculously, he did not contract the disease himself but lived on to fight other illnesses as a revered and respected physician.

His next past life memory was strongly linked both to his life in the Roman Empire and to the lifetime in France when he was a nun ministering to smallpox victims. Once more he was in the Middle Ages, at a somewhat earlier time, and again disease was rampant—a plague that affected most of Europe. He worked frantically, ministering to the overwhelming number of victims in the city where he lived (it might have been London; he wasn't sure), but his efforts were feeble against the pandemic. More than half of the citizens of the city died, as did his entire family. Exhausted by his struggles, he became despairing and bitter, and filled with guilt and remorse that he had failed so often. He could see ahead in that lifetime, telling me that he lived another ten years, but he never really forgave himself.

"Why were you so harsh with yourself?" I asked. "There was nothing you could do."

"Because I forgot about the bandages," he said from his superconscious state, floating above his Middle Ages body. "They could have kept away the fleas."

I was astonished. He had brought memories of an earlier past life into the Middle Ages! It was an indication of how closely his lives were linked and how all our past lives stay with us as we progress. Few people in the Middle Ages had the Romans' knowledge that fleas from infected rats spread the disease, but he felt he should have tapped into what he had learned in Rome and averted at least some of the deaths, perhaps saving his family as well.

He spoke again, still back with his medieval body. "I'll make you this promise. In all my future incarnations I'll protect and save as many people as I can. I know there is no death, that we're all immortal, but I'll do what I can to ease the pain of the victims and survivors to allow the soul's lessons to progress unimpeded."

He has kept his promise, I thought, in all but this life. What change would the memories inspire now? Would he find his true core as a healer?

We were both silent. I wondered fleetingly if David's presence was the harbinger of another epidemic—that seemed to be his pattern—and then shrugged off the thought as too fanciful. There was enough time left in the session to explore other lifetimes. I asked David whether he wanted to go to the past or the future.

His sadness vanished. "Oh, the future!"

He led me slightly more than one hundred years ahead in time. In that life the quintessential WASP who sat facing me was a rabbi!

"My name is Ephraim. I'm at a conference with Catholic, Protestant, Hindu, Buddhist, Muslim, holistic, and indigenous ministers and healers. We meet frequently, two or three times a week, to meditate and pray, creating a harmonious energy to combat the hate and violence endemic to the unenlightened inhabitants of the world. Our numbers are few, no more than fifty, but our power is great. Our purpose is to neutralize the Earth-damaging energies unknowingly unleashed by those who don't care or don't know about spiritual laws. Those energies create earthquakes, tornadoes, floods, epidemics. We used to think these were random events. Now we believe they're spawned—or at least influenced—by the thoughts and intentions of human-kind. And we can prevent them! Our group goes out to teach others the techniques of the positive prayer and positive meditation that we use. We have thousands of followers. Next month is our fifth ecumenical meeting of over twenty-five thousand who believe as we do; they will bring back our teachings to their own countries across the globe. These conferences transcend physical and psychological boundaries in order to achieve peace, harmony, and compassion for all the inhabitants of the world and for the planet itself."

His eyes were sparkling. "It's working! We're able to measure positive effects on the Earth's climate. The globe is cooling for the first time in centuries. Summers and winters are less severe. Cancer rates have gone down."

In one of his regressions David had alluded to the possibility of thought influencing natural phenomena. In this future he had apparently mastered the concept and made teaching it his life's work.

"I've learned how to teach others the way to invoke beings of higher consciousness," he confided in a tone of awe. (I thought of Sister Eugenie's past life experience.) "By communicating with a clear and compassionate heart, by seeking a higher spiritual good, we can solicit aid from them. They've already begun to help. The world is a far, far better place now than it was a hundred years ago."

David's gorgeous vision made me ponder. Whether the fruits of Ephraim's work will be realized in the actual future of the earth remains unclear. There are multiple futures open to us, some violent and some peaceful, and multiple paths to get to them. Certainly many other factors beyond his conferences and teachings will determine which becomes the actual one. My own feeling, however, is that the masters will play a role, and we would be wise, as David was, to listen to them. I had learned from many group progressions that several centuries from now a large decline in the Earth's population will occur. How this is effected, whether by war, disease, toxins, pole shifts (the Earth's axis changing), decline in fertility rate, conscious choice, or in unknown ways, has yet to be determined. I don't know whether Ephraim's mission succeeded in the end or whether the forces of violence, self-interest, greed, and hatred were just too powerful.

David was now observing Ephraim's life from a higher and more detached perspective. He seemed to know what I was thinking. "Whether the coming population decline is caused by traumatic events in a sudden and cataclysmic manner or whether it is gradual and more gentle in nature will be determined by the thoughts and actions of mankind. We all choose the lives we are about to lead. I chose well and helped others choose correctly, too. But were there enough of us, I wonder."

I wished I had more time with David to explore his issues further, but he had to go home to his pregnant wife and his family's business. I asked him to keep in touch with me, to let me know how the three sessions affected him, but I worried that the environment of comfort and ease in which he lived would seduce him again.

That did not happen. The knowledge of past and future lives helped David define his role in the present. He quit his father's firm and returned to Harvard to study environmental law. He felt he had to oppose the deleterious effects of certain big business practices—many of which his former firm defended—so that he could alter the future for the better. He was especially interested in issues of global warming, the careless accumulation of long-lived toxic by-products of industrial processes, and the resultant extinction of entire species of animals and plants without an understanding of what their absence would do to the balance of nature. At last, David is experiencing meaning and purpose in his life; he is "whole." His confusion has dissolved, and he is aligned with his destiny.

As David's story shows, spirituality does not reside in the mind alone but, rather, in one's entire persona, in the intentions and actions of a life lived well. You can't just think "I'm going to be spiritual from now on." You must also feel it as a consequence of your actions. We live in a community of souls, and we have to perform good deeds within that community. The introspective life is not by itself enough. When we reach out to assist fellow souls along their spiritual paths, we reach a higher level of evolution. David's past and future lifetimes demonstrate this altruistic devotion to loving service among his fellow humans. The more he gave, the more he received. Lives led spiritually, like his, bring us closer to our divine nature.

CHAPTER 13

Jennifer and Cristina:
Love

ANGER MANAGEMENT, health, empathy, compassion, patience
and understanding, nonviolence, relationships, security,
destiny and free will, contemplation and meditation, spirituality:
All these are steps to immortality. All these must be mastered now
or in the future in our journey to the one soul. And all these are
facets of the greatest virtue, which is love.

Love is the ultimate lesson. How can you retain anger if you
love? How can you not be compassionate or empathetic? How
can you not choose the right relationships? How can you strike
another? Foul the environment? War with a neighbor? Not have
room in your heart for other viewpoints, different methods, divergent lifestyles?

You can't.

When my patients have gone through regression and/or progression and have mastered their phobias and traumas, love is
what they understand. Many get this message from those who
play key roles in their lives. But many hear it from the other
side—from a parent, spouse, or child who has died. "I'm fine,"
the messages say. "I'm okay. I love you. You don't have to grieve

for me. What lies beyond is not darkness but light, for I am where love is, and love is light."

These messages might be wish fulfillment, fantasies to ease the pain of loss, but I don't think so. I've heard them too many times from too many people. Love is what we carry from life to life, although in some lifetimes we are unaware of it and in some misuse it. Ultimately, though, it is what keeps us evolving.

For example, Jennifer, having just given birth to her third child, was handed the baby for the first time. She recognized the child immediately—the energy, the expression in the eyes, the immediate connectedness. "You again," she said. "We're together again." The baby was the woman's grandmother in a past life. They had fought bitterly throughout that life, all the while loving each other, though the love went unexpressed. Now, she knew, was their chance to make amends.

There are all kinds of love, of course: romantic love; the love of a child for a parent and a parent for a child; and love of nature, of music, of poetry, of all things on this Earth and in the heavens. Love continues on the other side and is brought back here by the soul. It is the understanding of all the mysteries. To me it is the ultimate religion. If we could all love in our own way, if we could abandon the rituals that pronounce "Mine is the true path; all others are sham," if we could abjure the violence, conflicts, and pain we inflict in the name of a specific God—"our" God—when by definition God is universal, God is love, we would not have to wait through innumerable lifetimes to get to heaven.

Cristina dressed in a style that American women can't seem to emulate: flamenco-inspired skirts that reach the floor; blouses in bright reds, blues, purples, and yellows; luxuriant black hair pulled back severely and kept in place by ribbons of fantastic hues. When she first came to see me, I was struck by her showiness, but as her visits multiplied, I realized that the colors were compensation for her dark moods and darker thoughts. She was a woman fighting to retain a spark of self even as her family strove to snuff it out. There were dark patches of skin under her eyes, and her hands trembled slightly. Fatigue, I thought. She complained of asthma, and in times of stress it was apparent in her breathing, but it was her psychological problems that induced her to ask for my help.

Full-bodied but not fat, she exuded what turned out to be an ambiguous impression of strength within a palpable sexuality, and from the beginning she alternated between facing me squarely, almost hostilely, and averting her eyes from mine with a Latin demureness that bespoke a strict aristocratic upbringing. I guessed her to be in her late twenties; she turned out to be ten years older. She wore a ring on the fourth finger of her left hand, a large ruby that matched the flamboyance of her clothes, and I wondered if it was meant for decoration or as a proclamation of marriage.

"Divorced," she said, noting my look. "Two children. I wear the ring because it's beautiful and because it scares off suitors."

Her English was elegant, impeccable, yet I could detect traces of an accent. "You are not from Miami," I said—a statement, not a question.

"São Paulo, Brazil."

"Ah. And you moved here when?"

"Three years ago. To join my father after my divorce."

"You live with him, then?"

"No, no. He lives with my mother in Bal Harbour. I'm a few miles away."

"With your children?"

"Yes. The girls. Rosana is seven, Regina five. They're very dear."

"So when you say you came to join your father—"

"To work with him. To be with him in his business."

"Which is what?"

"Really? You don't know? I went back to my maiden name after the divorce, and I'd have thought you'd recognize it."

Of course! Stupid of me. I should have made the connection immediately. Her father was head of a company specializing in high-end clothing. In the past two years it had branched out into a line of younger, less expensive sportswear, which my wife, Carole, later told me was once *the* thing to wear if you were a teenager. I asked if Cristina's move coincided with her father's new venture.

"Coincidental," she said. "I make no decisions and have no say in planning." Her eyes flashed with anger. "I'm little more than a servant girl with her own office."

"And this is frustrating to you?"

"Frustrating? It's *infuriating!*" She leaned toward me and spoke with passion that made her tremble. "My God, what I could do if he let me! He makes clothes for women but doesn't believe women should have the final say in how they look. My eye is twice as good as his. I'm twice as clever. His clothes were a fad, and like all fads, they became obsolete. Already people have stopped buying. My clothes would be timeless."

Cristina, I thought, could accomplish whatever she set out to do. "But he won't listen?" I asked.

"He shuts me off like a car engine. I've given up trying. To fight him is like fighting an army of the Inquisition."

"What about your mother? Can she help?"

"She can't help herself. My mother's simply a decoration, like a vase of flowers. She shuts up because she knows he could replace her whenever he felt like it."

"But he hasn't."

"Sure he has, a million times. He keeps his women in separate apartments or separate hotels, depending on how serious he feels about them. In his religion divorce is not allowed. I defied it and divorced four years ago. He almost killed me when I did; it's only when he knew he needed me that he let me come to America."

"Does your mother know about the other women?"

"She'd be a fool if she didn't." Cristina paused. "But then, she *is* a fool!"

I did not remark on her bitterness. "Are you an only child?"

"Only daughter. I have two older brothers."

"Do they work in the business, too?"

"Work is the wrong word. They come into the office and go out to lunch."

"Yet they get the promotions, the respect. They're listened to." It was an easy guess.

"My father is too savvy to take their advice. But you're right about the promotions and the respect. You see, I'm a woman and deserve neither."

It was a familiar complaint of Latin women, stifled by a culture that had not progressed into the twentieth century. She was obviously the star of the family, yet she was obscured by the cloud of tradition and closed-mindedness.

"Why don't you leave, strike out on your own?"

It was as though I had accused her of murder. Ashen-faced, she pushed back from her chair, stood, and then collapsed back down. She began to cry, dissolving under what seemed to me an obvious question. "I don't know," she wailed, all sophistication gone, suddenly defenseless. "Please, *please*. I need your help!"

The change in her was so sudden that beyond a mumbled "Of course I'll help," I felt awed. "Tell me the problem," I said. "Be as precise as you can."

She looked at me through tear-filled eyes and breathed with difficulty. "You have to understand one thing: I love my father. No matter what I tell you, that's the underlying truth."

Love him and hate him, I thought. Hardly a unique emotional conflict.

"When he came to America, leaving me and my husband and babies behind, I felt relieved. My brothers went with him, and it seemed that by their going, I was rid of all the constraints, all the pressures imposed on me by a tyrannical Brazilian patriarch of the old school." She laughed ruefully. "Men a thousand, women zero. He never hit me, never was cruel. On the contrary, he gave me everything I wanted, and that was the trouble. I never *earned* them—or, rather, I earned them by being obedient. When I was still a little girl, I realized I was smarter than my brothers. By the time I was twenty, I knew I was smarter than my father, too. I worked for him for a while in Brazil, helped the company grow— *really* helped—without taking any credit for it. But it didn't do me any good. I was diminished, shunted aside, not only by him but by my brothers who were jealous of my brains and my mother who was his slave. It wasn't right. It wasn't just. So I married the first man who came after me without realizing he was just as tyrannical—and *he* hit."

By now the tears had stopped. Her voice was level, though I could feel the intense emotion behind her words. I had no doubt that she was reporting accurately. Cristina was a woman pitted against an age-old culture with age-old beliefs, and as strong as she was, they had bested her.

She took a deep breath. "Okay. My family's in Miami, *he's* in Miami, and I'm in São Paulo with a terrible husband and two babies I adore. My father opposes my divorce, but I go through with it anyway. I had no choice; he was hitting the girls, too. And only when it's final do I tell Father. From him, silence. Many months, silence.

"And then all of a sudden he calls. 'Come to Miami. Work with me in the company. You're alone. I'll take care of you.' So I came. I thought he was taking pity on me—generosity and compassion from a man who had never shown them. The line for teenagers was my idea, and I was thrilled when we began to work together again. I fed him other ideas. He ate them like chocolates. But pretty soon I realized nothing had changed, that he was using me, that my brothers were the beneficiaries of my talent—that he was a greedy, self-serving, cold-blooded villain."

"And yet," I pointed out, "you say you love him."

The thought crossed my mind that he might have abused her sexually when she was young, but I dismissed it; she exhibited none of the symptoms. No, the abuse was psychological. By putting her under his domination, he created a kind of Stockholm syndrome in her soul wherein the captive falls in love with the captor. He tormented her, but there was no one she could turn to, no one she could trust. It was the most insidious kind of sadism. She had no choice but to love him.

She seemed exhausted by her narrative, and I asked her if she wanted to rest. No, she said, it was better to get the whole story out. "I struck out on my own. I moved me and the children out of the house to where I live now and told him I was going to start my own line of clothes."

"Did he get angry?" I asked, visualizing his rage.

"Worse. He laughed. He told me I'd never get financing, that nobody would give money to a *woman*. He said if I did manage to start a business of my own, he'd disinherit me and the girls. 'You can walk the streets for all I care' is what he said. But I went ahead anyway. About a year ago I quit his company, wrote my own marketing plan for another, and rented an office. I talked to wholesalers and retail buyers."

"Without any money?"

"Well, I'd saved my salary when I lived at home, and I got a small business loan from the bank. But I didn't have nearly enough, even with the loan, and these first months have been tough going. Still, I made a few sales. The buyer for Bloomingdale's in Miami bought my line of office wear. She said I had accomplished 'miracles' in a short time. I was on my way. Of course, when my father found out about it, he stopped speaking to me. I had hope for my new life, but the anxiety is tremendous. I have nightmares, so I'm afraid to sleep. I shout at my children. I'm eating out of nervousness. I've gained ten pounds, all on junk food. My breathing gets so bad, I sometimes think I'm going to die."

"You say you 'had' hope. Has it gone?"

She bowed her head. "Yes."

"Do you know why?"

Again she dissolved, and she gasped out her answer through her tears. "My father has asked me to come back."

His company was going bankrupt. With all its fame and despite the fact that stores were filled with his merchandise, he was in deep financial trouble. Although his up-market clothes still sold—it was his strength in that area which accounted for his initial rise—the lower-end part of the business was failing. Cristina was right when she said customers had stopped buying. Orders for the following year were down 40 percent, a calamitous decline.

"He's on the verge of bankruptcy," Cristina said after she had explained the facts, "and he's asked me to come back and save him."

"And that's why you've come to see me?"

"Yes. Because I can't make up my mind about what to do, and it's driving me crazy."

"Oh, you're not crazy," I assured her, "just stuck. Sometimes when decisions are monumental, it prevents us from making them at all."

She looked at me gratefully. Although what I had said was neither profound nor original, I had pinpointed the problem. "Maybe it will help if we go through your options."

"Good," she said, her composure regained. Her words came quickly now. She had already sorted through the choices in her mind. "First, I can go back to my father and help him as he has asked. That would mean giving up my life for him, a kind of suicide for a family cause. Second, I can stop working and remarry. I'd choose carefully this time. This time it would be for love—and have more children, like millions of my sisters around the world. My parents would approve, my culture would thank me, and I suppose I could make myself a happy but unfulfilled life."

She paused, obviously visualizing it, and shook her head sadly. "Or I could go on with my own clothing line." She brightened. "It would work, you know. Dr. Weiss, I didn't tell you this before, but when it comes to business decisions, I'm psychic. Don't smile. Really. I *know* I'd succeed. It's only in life decisions that I mess up."

Many successful business people have Cristina's gift. They call it "gut instinct" or "flying by the seat of their pants" or "playing a hunch," but it is actually a kind of psychic power. Again, I didn't doubt that Cristina possessed it, and it seemed to point to the right path.

"What's the downside?" I asked.

She sighed. "Many. Compete with him in his own business? My family has cast me out already, even my mother, and if I go on, they'll never forgive me. Frankly, I don't know if I could forgive myself. It's such a betrayal of them—of him—that I'd feel I deserved his anger and any punishment that came with it."

"But isn't that what you're doing now? Competing with him?"

"Absolutely. And that's what has made it so hard to sleep and filled me with such anxiety." She saw my surprised expression. "Oh, it isn't the *business* part of it that worries me. I've already performed miracles, as the Bloomingdale's buyer said. I told you I'm psychic. It's that if he goes bankrupt, my success would literally kill him."

"I don't understand, then, why you started your own business at all."

"Because I was angry. Because he betrayed me, and I wanted revenge. Because—" Here she stopped, and the tears started. "I don't think I could have gone on with my business. When it was successful, I think I'd have given it to him. Actually, some great part of me didn't want it to succeed. I'd already planned to give it up before I came to see you."

"There are a number of factors here," I said sympathetically. "You've been betrayed, but you will feel guilty if you strike back. You're angry, but you're afraid of the consequences. You're psychic, but you can't figure out the future. Men have only hurt you, but you're willing to remarry. You love and hate your father simultaneously. Does that sum it up?"

She laughed despite herself. "Tell me, Doctor, what are my chances?"

"We must see if we can look into the future," I said. "But to do that, let's go to your past."

Her first regression was a short one. All she could tell me was that she lived in an Islamic culture of North Africa; she couldn't place the date or describe her surroundings. She knew that she was male, a writer of verse, and that she had a father, also a writer, of whom she was extremely jealous, for he outshone his son in recognition, prominence, and income. The parallels to her present life were so direct and obvious that she felt what she saw might have been nothing more than a fantasy.

The second regression was more interesting.

"It's the Middle Ages. Twelfth century. I'm a young man, a priest, very handsome, living in the mountains—it looks like south-central France. There are deep gorges and valleys, so traveling is difficult, but many people come to me. They are in need of my ability to give physical and psychological succor. I believe in reincarnation and inspire others to believe in it also, which is a great comfort to them. People who are diseased—lepers and sick children—seek me out, and when I touch them, many of them are miraculously cured. Of course I am a beloved figure. No one else has my talent.

"My father in my present life is a farmer in this one, and he lives not a mile away. He's everything I'm not: greedy, godless, acquisitive, a misanthrope. He's the richest man in the region, but his money and land don't tempt the free-spirited village girl he covets, though he would give them all for her love. She loves me and is willing to accept only spiritual, platonic love, for I am true to my vows of celibacy. 'By loving you I show my love for God,' she tells me.

"An invading army from Rome has been able to ford the gorges and has surrounded the village. They attack. I am captured. The farmer denounces me to the authorities, claiming I practice black magic. When they hear stories of my power to heal and my certainty of lives to come, they believe the farmer, and I am burned at the stake. It's an agonizing death, for along with the flames, the smoke makes it impossible to see my beloved who, weeping, has come to watch me die and to give whatever solace she can. Moments after I die, she hurls herself down a gorge and is killed instantly.

"In death I am able to look down at the village to see what transpires. The farmer's jealousy of me, which I barely recognized when I was alive, never disappears. He has to settle for a loveless marriage and grows more bitter, more cruel. In my life review I can see myself come back in a future life to help the farmer, now a blacksmith, with his life lessons, but I am not able to give him much help. He will come back again and again without progress. I feel I've failed, and I've failed because deep in my Christian heart I hate him. He killed me and, worse, the woman I loved. I rejoice that he was bitter, unfulfilled, and miserable. I know my thoughts are wrong, but I can't help it. It would be a lie to pretend anything else."

When Cristina left that day, I made a note to see if her asthma got better, for I felt that the priest's death by fire and smoke was linked to it. (This is fairly common; breathing problems often have past-life causes.) In fact, it was markedly improved by our next session and is not nearly as debilitating today.

I made another note: "Jealousy is what hooked farmer and priest together in another life and probably in this one. In this life, Cristina's father was presented with the opportunity to redeem himself for the jealousy and treachery he displayed toward her in past lives. He could have supported her psychologically by recognizing and acknowledging her talent, and he could have rewarded her by promoting her in the company. He chose to do neither. Perhaps yet another lifetime will be needed for him to learn compassion and altruism."

In her next and last regression Cristina found herself in a small town in England in the 1800s.

"It's an exciting place to be," she told me. "For the first time in history, men are going off to work, leaving their houses to go to offices or factories, while women are put in sole charge of the home. It means a new kind of society, different relationships between husband and wife. But I'm lucky: I'm still young, twenty, not married, and have taken a job in a textile plant so I can make some money. Once I get there, I think of all sorts of ways to increase production and reduce costs simultaneously. My supervisor is impressed and asks my advice all the time. He's terrifically handsome, and he says he loves me. I sure love him."

The supervisor in that life was once again her father in this one. I led her forward in her past life, noting a marked change in her expression. She was no longer a happy, carefree girl but a bitter, disillusioned woman. The supervisor, it turns out, betrayed her.

"He didn't love me after all. He pretended to so he could steal my ideas and take them as his own. He was promoted. His superiors called him a genius. Oh, it's horrible! I *hate* him! One day I confronted him in front of his boss and begged him to confess that 'his' ideas were really mine. The next day he accused me of stealing five pounds from a coworker. I was innocent, totally innocent, but the girl backed him up. She was probably his mistress, and he told her he loved her so she would take his side. It'll serve her right when she finds out what a bastard he is. I was arrested, sent to prison for a year, humiliated, and abandoned. In jail I developed pneumonia. It didn't kill me, but it weakened my lungs, and I had coughing spells for the rest of my life." (Another parallel with her present-day asthma.) "I couldn't get another job but was forced to beg. I had promise, real promise—all my coworkers at the factory thought so—but what good did it do me? It destroyed me." She began to cry.

"Did you ever forgive him?" I asked.

"Never! Hatred of him was the fuel that kept me going. 'I'll see him dead before I die,' I told myself. But it was a promise I couldn't keep. I died before I was forty, unmarried, childless, alone. He probably lived to be a hundred. What injustice! What a waste of my life on this Earth."

Not really. The tragedy of that past life and of her life as a priest was preparation for this life and her lives to come. When I brought her back to the present, she remained in an altered state that I could not precisely define.

"The Bible tells us that the sins of the father carry on to the third or fourth generation of descendants." (I looked it up. She was paraphrasing Exodus 20:5.) "But that doesn't make sense. We are our own descendants, reincarnated as our grandchildren, great-grandchildren, and great-great-grandchildren throughout our many lives. And at any point we can *erase* those sins, because they don't exist in another, they exist in ourselves. My father was in all my lives. I recognized him as my father, a farmer, a supervisor. And in each life I've loved him, then hated him. His sins have followed him down through the centuries."

She leaned forward, inspired. "But so have mine. It wasn't—isn't—his sins I must change. It's my own. I've hated him for millennia. Hatred is a sin. Each time that hatred eradicated the love I felt for him at the beginning. But what if it's different this time? What if I can eradicate hatred with love?"

Cristina's extraordinary insights did not, of course, answer the question of which choice to make—employee, housewife, or competitor—in the next months. At the time of our working together I was just beginning my progression work and was using it selectively. Cristina's strength and intellect made her an excellent candidate, I thought, and I suggested we try going forward.

She agreed readily. "We're only going to look at possible futures pertaining to your choices," I told her. "I want to avoid glimpses of serious illness, loss, or death. If you find yourself going in that direction, tell me, and I'll bring you back."

I started by asking her to see herself if she had stayed in her father's company. "I'm sick, physically sick," she said at once, but despite my admonition, she stopped me from bringing her back. "It's a sickness born of frustration. The job is stifling me literally and figuratively. My asthma is worse. I can't breathe. It's like being in England two centuries ago. I'm in prison."

Her vision of herself as a housewife was equally bleak. "My children are both grown and have moved away. I'm alone. I never remarried. My head feels empty, like my brain has shriveled up from lack of use. I see my inventiveness as belonging to other lives, not this one."

As for starting a competitive business: "I'm successful. My father is bankrupt, and I'm a multimillionaire. Nevertheless, I'm miserable. It all feels angry and vindictive. I've lost by winning. My family and I never see each other, never speak. We sit in our rooms, separated by silence, spending our days with hatred."

When I brought her back, I expected sadness. Instead, jubilation!

"There is a fourth choice," she cried, "one I didn't see before: Start my own business but not in competition with my father."

"Won't that be risky?" I asked.

"I don't think so. Marketing and design skills apply to all businesses. Cookware! Ceramics! I'm a good cook and an okay potter, so at least I'll know what I'm talking about, though naturally I'll get expert advice. I have an in with the stores that might sell them and a record with my present start-up that's the equal of anybody's. I'll go back to the lenders who helped me get started and tell them I've changed my plans, but not to worry. I'll come up with a new marketing plan, a new business plan—I'm an expert at those. I'll design stockpots, casseroles, coffee cups, dinner services. I'll work with clay, with steel, with silver. And nobody will say I'm out to beat my father. Why, when it succeeds, he'll be proud of me and love me at last."

Her enthusiasm was so boundless that I didn't have the heart to point out the pitfalls. I was sure she would succeed—but win her father's love? Something profound would have to change in both of them before that was possible.

She left effusing gratitude, but I remained unsatisfied. True, I had helped her solve her dilemma, but there was more work to be done. I thought back to her insight about the transmission of sin and wondered if she would take it further. I was therefore pleased when a few months later she called for an appointment.

She had had rocky going, she told me. Her new plans were not met with the support she had expected. She had yet to find her own "design voice." She had had to change her children's school from private to public. She was worried about money, afraid she'd have to go back to her father after all, if only to support her children. Yet she described her problems with an ebullience lacking in her earlier visits; the darkness under her eyes had also disappeared, and she breathed far more easily. I pointed this out and asked her why.

"I'm in love."

I was astonished. When she left, I figured it would be a long time before she would let love in—she was too angry at men, too determined to be alone—yet there was no mistaking the light in her eyes.

"Tell me."

"Ricardo's wonderful. Won-der-ful! I met him at a reading group. We discovered that we share a love for *Don Quixote,* maybe because we both tilt at windmills. He's a commercial flier, a freelancer who hires out to international companies operating between here and Latin America. He's been to São Paulo and even knows the street where I lived. He speaks Spanish and Portuguese, and when I told him about you, he said he'd read one of your books in Portuguese when he was last in Brazil because he couldn't get the English-language edition. It was your first one, he thinks, the one about you and your patient—I've forgotten the title, too—though I'm afraid he doesn't believe all of it. Do you mind?"

"Of course not. I'm glad you're happy. But I'm surprised, really, that you're in love."

She looked at me with enormous gravity. "I'm surprised, too. I asked myself how it could happen, and so suddenly, and I believe I have the answer. It's because of what we talked about earlier. The moment I realized I was a sinner as well as my father and that my sin is hate, as it has been through all my past lives, then my hatred of him, of all men, vanished—and into my life walked Ricardo. I know it sounds all too pat, but it's true!"

She put her hands on my desk and leaned toward me. "It's the strangest thing, Dr. Weiss. When I look at him, *really* look, I see the good part of my soul. He's me, I know, and I'm him. But it seems impossible."

I explained that when a soul is fragmented from the One, it can enter more than one body simultaneously and that her feeling wasn't "strange" or even particularly unusual. She and Ricardo were destined to meet, I told her, and now their free choice would determine what would happen to them in the future.

"I have an idea of what that might be," she said, smiling radiantly.

So did I.

There remained the question of whether her new business would succeed or fail. I asked her if she wanted me to lead her into the future, and after considerable hesitation—in her current euphoria, she didn't want bad news—she agreed. Only instead of going a few years forward, she went twelve hundred! Usually when people progress into the distant future, they're not sure of the year, but Cristina was positive: 3200.

"The earth is very green," she said, "much greener and more fertile than it is now. The forests are lush, the meadows filled with flowers. But funnily enough there are no animals. Why, when there's so much food for them to eat? There aren't many people, either. They can communicate with one another telepathically, and their bodies, less dense than ours, are filled with light. They live in small groups, not cities, in lovely houses made of wood or stone, and they seem to be farmers. I can see liquid or liquid light pouring into the plants; sometimes the liquid pours into the people themselves. The people are extremely spiritual. I can't see any illness, any real anger, or any violence or war. There's a certain translucent quality to everything, a permeating light that connects everyone and everything in peace."

"How did it make you feel, seeing the world this way?" I asked when I had brought her back to the present.

She beamed. "Calm. Comfortable. Joyous. I look forward to living there."

"I wonder why you went there instead of the immediate future."

She considered the question. "Because it's more important. I can handle the years in this life by myself. My business will flourish like the trees and plants two millennia from now. With Ricardo to love, how can it fail?"

She was right, of course. Within eighteen months her goods were in upscale stores across the country, and when Carole and I went to Russia, we saw them in St. Petersburg. She was also doing a burgeoning business on the Internet. She invested some of her profits in her father's business and saved him from the threatened bankruptcy. Ricardo and she married, and I pretty much lost contact with her. But one morning she called me. I could hear the elation in her voice.

"I had to tell you, Dr. Weiss, because it's thanks to you that it happened. Last night Ricardo and I were at my parents' for dinner. We go often; they like him. Anyway, as we were leaving, my father drew me aside and hugged me. *Hugged me!* It felt wonderful. And then for the first time in my life or his, he told me that he loved me."

Love is an absolute quality and energy. It does not stop with our death. It continues on to the other side and returns here again. It is the epitome of the spirit's quality—and the body's. It is life and the afterlife. It is our goal, and all of us, in this or future lives, will attain it.

CHAPTER 14

Gary:
The Future

I N ALL MY BOOKS I've tried to convey the astonishing impact of the regression sessions; the effect of the "miraculous" visions, not only physically but psychically; the sense of mystery or magic or transcendence that both the patient and I experience. How much more wondrous is it then when we travel to the future to see not what has happened but what *will* happen, what will be. Such journeys continue to fill me with awe and caution. I'm wary of leading my patients to realms that might be imaginary and have them base their life decisions on what they "see," and I stress to them the danger of illusion or fantasy.

One caveat when conceptualizing about the future is the possibility of projecting one's own subconscious wishes to create future scenarios. For a psychoanalyst such scenarios are vitally important because whatever the deeper mind creates is grist for the therapeutic mill and is significant to the creator. In this sense, future memories are like dreams. There is often a mixture of symbol and metaphor, deep-seated hopes and wishes, actual memories and precognitive experiences. In other words, just because a patient sees the future doesn't mean that it is a "real" future. Nevertheless, the immediacy and strength of the memories can instantly improve the present and future course of the patient's life. To a therapist these changes are even more important than the capacity to validate the material.

Still, many near future visions have proven true; you've seen the results in several of the cases in this book. And if we learn to infallibly distinguish between truth and fantasy, something that will probably not happen in this generation but perhaps the next, then all of us who see into the future, whether we use the material therapeutically or not, can improve that future by improving ourselves. And the golden immortality that is ours eventually will arrive more quickly, and we will traverse verdant fields and shining sky to the One.

I believe we can see the future because some part of us responds to the fact that past, present, and future are one, occurring in a simultaneous time, quite different from the longitudinal years, months, days, hours, and minutes by which we measure time on Earth. Quite literally the future *is* now, and even on this planet we can shape our "nows" by our actions. That is why it is so important to prepare not only for the rest of our lives but for all our lives to come—for immortality.

The future seems to be a flexible destination. There exists a multitude of possible futures and probable futures across a vast statistical spectrum. Our *individual* immediate futures in this life and those shortly to come depend to a large extent, as we have seen, on our choices and actions in the present. Our long-term futures—our *collective* futures, the future of our planet (which may exist forever but which we may destroy, though by destroying it we will not stop our progress toward the One)—depend on the cumulative decisions of all people. What those decisions are can be seen in the view of the future some one thousand years from now. The closer we get to a particular future, the more accurate we can be in predicting it. It is important to look one thousand years and more ahead because the Earth today is becoming dangerous, and perhaps if we apply more wisdom to our decisions because of what we see, we can alter the direction of the future starting now.

When I work with the groups who attend my seminars, I progress them into the distant future, into discrete time periods: one hundred years from now, five hundred years, one thousand years or more. I want to see if there is agreement in the visions, for if they match, there is a good chance there is truth in them, that the world will look and feel much as they foretell. My experiments are still young, but I have found such striking similarities in 90 percent of them that more and more I have come to believe there is an excellent chance, scores of lifetimes hence, that a glorious world awaits us.

I use individual progressions for therapy. As I noted, I did so only recently and with some reluctance, for I was concerned about self-fulfilling prophecy in the unstable patient. Still, some of my patients were spontaneously going into the future anyway and benefiting from it, and I began to use the technique, leading patients near to their deaths without letting them actually view it. If we see the end of our lives, perhaps there are three or four more steps we can take now, more choices we can opt for, as we proceed toward the next life. (Some people overrode my therapeutic suggestion and went to their actual deaths, but they were strong enough to handle it; those that weren't strong invariably didn't.)

I found that people made wiser decisions and better choices when they saw ahead. They looked at the forks in the road and said, "If I take this path, this path, this path, or this path, what would be the differences?" As we make choices now, we're constantly changing our futures. But overall, out of the infinity of futures that face us, there are one or more *probable* futures, and maybe we have a 5 percent chance of going this way, a 10 percent chance of going another, and only a .0001 percent chance of a third. It is a system of probabilities and possibilities that we're constantly altering. Remember that all our individual futures are

part of a universal arc; when those myriad individual futures coalesce with the higher spirit in the far future, we will reach our
goal.

For now it is the choices that matter. John, for example, saw a
fork in the road that determined a compassionate present life,
hugely different from the one he was currently leading. Evelyn
saw a future where her deep-seated hatred no longer existed, and
she was able to begin her path to that state in the present. When
we see the future, it doesn't mean that we're forced into it—hence
the forks in so many instances. There are still choices, and it's not
too late to make them.

In both John's and Evelyn's cases, and in the others I've
already described, we regressed before we went ahead. Going forward without going back was essential in Gary's therapy, however, for he came to me in crisis. The night before he called, he
had had a dream of himself pointing a gun at his own head, his
finger slowly pulling the trigger. It seemed appropriate, he told
me when he described it after I had taken his history. Death
would mean the end of despair.

Gary was a physically healthy man of forty whose antiques business was about to collapse. Because of the success of *Antiques
Roadshow* on television, he assumed that a rage for high-priced
silver, paintings, and furniture would sweep the nation, so he ex-
panded his inventory to the point where he had to rent an extra
warehouse to contain it. But either because his taste was poor or
because he had overestimated the market, he attracted few additional buyers. When the loans he had taken to buy the stock came
due, he couldn't pay them. His partner sued him for mismanage-
ment of funds. He had to fire his staff. His children, twin boys,
were about to enter college, and he couldn't pay their tuition. His
adored wife, Constance, had just been diagnosed with multiple
sclerosis. A lawyer suggested he file for bankruptcy, but to Gary
the idea was unthinkable.

He told me all this in a rush, his gaunt face drawn and gray, his eyes filled with sorrow. "Hence the dream," he said. "You can see why it was so powerful."

"Why is the idea of bankruptcy unthinkable?" I asked. "It seems to me the only reasonable solution."

"Because it proves my father right."

"About what?"

" 'My boy, you'll never amount to anything.' If he said it once, he said it a thousand times."

"He's deceased?"

"For twelve years."

"But you remember his words."

"I'm haunted by them. My father was a strong man, Dr. Weiss. My mother died when I was three, and he brought me up alone. He was a construction worker, a hard hat, but he never went out drinking with his buddies, never found another woman—didn't look for one—never did anything save care for me, worry about me, save his money for me. By God, he said, I'd be the first in my family to go to college. He wanted me to be a lawyer or a doctor or a scientist. I'd make him proud.

"I tried, really I did, but I couldn't master math or chemistry or physics, and my mind just isn't logical. I could no more be a lawyer than a construction worker."

"It doesn't take a logical mind to be a construction worker."

"No, but it takes strength." He stood and spread his arms. "Look at me."

What I saw was an ordinary man who could be described as "average build, average height." It wasn't his self that prevented him from physical work, it was his self-image.

"I was interested in art," he continued, "Egyptian, Greek, Roman, Renaissance. In my sophomore year at Tulane I decided to major in art history, but it wasn't until my junior year that I told my father."

"What happened?"

His lips curled in rage. " 'My boy, you'll never amount to anything.' He called me a sissy, a pansy, an *intellectual*—there could be nothing worse. I had betrayed him, shattered his hopes, was proof he had wasted his life. 'I wish I'd had a girl,' he said. To him being a girl was almost as bad as being an intellectual."

"Did he disown you?"

"Worse. He kept paying my tuition, my room and board. He said he had nothing else to do with his money, that he was too old to start a life. When I came home for summers and holidays, he was cordial. *Cordial,* as though I was a stranger, which I suppose I was. After I started my business, I tried to pay him back, but he tore up the first check I handed him, and I never tried again. Making me guilty was his revenge, and he succeeded at it."

"You were under terrific pressure," I said. "It's hard to pretend to be something you're not, even harder to be despised for who you are." His look of self-pity was testament to the truth of this. "But you made a life for yourself. Many others with fathers like yours couldn't have done that."

"Some achievement," he said bitterly. "Face it: I'm a failure."

"Business failure is no disgrace. Happens all the time. You'll pull out of it. Meanwhile, you have a wife who loves you—"

"Who *says* she does."

I was struck by the emphasis in his words. "You don't think it's true?"

He was utterly despondent. "How could it be?"

He was in such despair that I felt it useless to point out that she must have loved him when she married him, and she almost surely loved him still, or at least that part of him that had attracted her in the first place. "What's the major sign that she doesn't love you?"

A wildness came into his expression.

"When I told her I wanted to kill myself, she begged me not to."

I was momentarily stunned. "That proves she *doesn't* love you?" I said at last.

"If she did, she'd let me do it." He gave a strange little laugh.

"But it doesn't matter. I'll do it no matter how hard she tries to stop me."

"When?"

"How about tomorrow? That suit you? It suits me fine."

Threats of suicide are among the most serious issues a psychiatrist faces. That Gary had come to see me meant at the very least that he was ambivalent about his decision, that his dream had scared him. Perhaps he was merely trying to shock me or dramatize himself. The degree of misery, however, argued that the desire was there, and I knew I could take no chances.

"I'll have to hospitalize you."

He stared at me, eyes suddenly devoid of all expression. "No way."

"You're in danger of dying."

"It's not a danger, it's a resolution."

"Not by anyone except you. You already told me your wife has tried to stop you. I'll bet your boys would try to stop you, too."

"The boys are away."

"Then think of their shock, of their grief."

"They'd say they were well rid of me. They think I'm worthless, and they're right. They'd be better off without me."

Again, argument seemed futile. If I couldn't shake him from his wish, then I would have to hospitalize him. But if I could get him to reach a higher perspective and to visualize the consequence of his suicide . . . "I'll make a deal with you."

He seemed startled. "What deal?"

"If you spend two sessions with me, letting me try to help you, I won't hospitalize you."

"And if I still feel the same way after the sessions, you won't try to stop me?"

That couldn't, of course, be part of the deal. "Let's just see what we can achieve," I said. "I want you to visit the future."

* * *

When Gary was under deep hypnosis, I instructed him to look at the two paths diverging from his place in the present. One path would show him the aftereffects of his suicide. The other was the path of positive action, love of self, and life.

We chose to look first at the path of suicide. Immediately, his eyes filled with tears.

"I was wrong. Constance did love me. I see her grieving, and it is many years after my death. The boys are grieving, too. I was so selfish that I didn't even consider them when I pulled the trigger. But they had to leave college and look after Constance in her illness." He paused, and when he spoke again, it was with a tone of amazement. "The funny thing is, they all feel responsible for my death. Their guilt is consuming them. They think they could have protected me from myself, saved me if they had been more diligent. I can't believe it! It was my hand, not theirs, on the gun. And Constance had done all she could. She pleaded with me. I didn't believe her, and I went ahead."

"Their reaction isn't so strange," I said quietly. "In many cases the survivors feel responsible."

His tears began to fall. "Oh, I'm sorry about that. So, so sorry. I didn't mean—"

"To hurt them?"

"Yes. *I* was the one in pain."

Suicide is not an act of altruism. It is an act of anger or despair. I would point this out to Gary when I brought him back, but it was important for him to know more about the future. I led him even further, into his next life.

His fingers gripped the sides of his chair until the knuckles were white. "There's a man standing, holding a gun at his head. I can see his finger tightening on the trigger."

"Is the man you?"

"Yes!"

"With the gun to your head, as it was in the dream you reported when you first came to see me?"

His body relaxed. "A dream. Yes. That's what it is. A dream."

"Does it mean you want to kill yourself?"

"Yes. I deserve to die. I've been having an affair."

"So you're married?"

"Of course. And I work for my father-in-law."

"An affair doesn't seem a reason for suicide."

"You don't understand. If my wife finds out, she'll tell her father, and I'll lose everything: job, family, position, my friends, my self-esteem. I couldn't stand the humiliation."

"The affair is secret. Why does your wife have to know?"

"Because my lover has written her a letter telling her everything. I've broken up with her, you see, and she's gone crazy. The letter is her revenge."

"But the affair is over. You ended it. Why not just admit it and apologize to your wife before she gets the letter? In time she'd forgive you. Maybe she wouldn't tell her father."

"Not a chance. She never loved me as much as she loves him. In fact, I don't think she loved me at all."

"So she'll be glad if you kill yourself?"

"There'll be a celebration. She'll invite her father and her friends."

His bitterness was as deep as it was in the present. "Does the dream seem familiar?" I asked.

The question startled him. He thought for a while and then said hesitantly, "You mean like a recurrent dream? No, I don't think so. Only . . ." He shook his head. "No."

"Did you in fact kill yourself?"

He frowned. There was another silence. Finally: "I don't know. I can't see. Oh, God! *I don't know what to do.*"

He remembered his future dream in his present life when he came back to it. "Does this mean I'll have the old feelings, the humiliation and the despair, over and over again?"

"Is that what it feels like?"

"It seems I'll want to kill myself forever. That no matter my life, that's the pattern it'll take."

"Until you're ready to learn," I agreed. "It's like a Greek tragedy. If you kill yourself now, you're destined to face the situation over and over again. What you failed to realize was that the man in your dream and the man you saw in your progression—the man with the gun at his head—wasn't actually you but only a part of you, the self-loathing part, the suicidal part."

He shuddered as though suddenly chilled. "If I took the other road," he said, "what would that be like?"

"Ah, good question. It's there you'll be able to learn."

It took longer than usual for him to be hypnotized, perhaps because he was fearful that the second path, too, would lead to despair. But at length he found himself in the near future, having chosen not to kill himself after all.

"I did go into bankruptcy," he reported, "but I won the lawsuit. There were really no grounds for it."

"And Constance?"

"Totally supportive. So were the kids. So were my friends. I think they felt that all of us make mistakes, and they forgave me for mine. In fact, they didn't feel I needed forgiveness. I was their husband and their father and their friend, not infallible, not God."

"How did you cope financially?"

"We sold the house and got a smaller one. I was able to pay off my outstanding debts, to say nothing of the medical bills."

"The boys?"

"Stayed in school. They had to bunk in the same room when they came home, but they didn't seem to mind."

"What's your work now?"

He smiled. "Rare coins. They were a hobby of mine, and now they're my vocation."

"Doing well?"

"Splendidly, thank you. I've hired back some of the people I had to let go. They were happy to come and even left jobs to join me. I guess they didn't think I was a bad boss or a failure. I'd told them the truth when I fired them. One of them said he admired my honesty and compassion. Of course, my antiques business also started well, so who knows?"

I progressed him further, toward the end of his life. "There are grandchildren," he said. "My Constance died many years ago, but I was able to comfort her in her last days, and we continued to love each other until the end." He sighed. "It's been a good life, all in all."

I knew, given his change of heart and mind, that his next one would be better. In it, Gary was a scientist doing research in plant physiology—specifically, creating species that were nutritionally complete so that people could healthily embrace vegetarianism as an alternative to eating animals of higher consciousness. There was no business scenario at all, no adultery, no despondency, not a glimmer of a thought of suicide.

There was no question as to which path he would choose when I brought him back to the present. He would avoid the first path, he realized, because he could choose wisely in the present. Indeed, Gary's life is thus far developing exactly as he had foreseen in the life path he had chosen. His family has continued to love and support him. He won his lawsuit. He has started a new business, a gallery for modern artists (one's visions of the future are rarely 100 percent accurate), and new drugs have relieved some of Constance's symptoms, though both are resigned to the reality of her disease. A few days ago he called me with some news: One of his sons had decided to leave college to become a rock musician.

"What do you think about it?" I asked.

"I hate it."

"What did you tell him?"

"I said, 'My boy, you'll amount to something no matter what you decide to do.' "

* * *

While I believe there are forks in all our lives and that progression into the future can help us decide which path to take, I also believe that there are forks in the life of the world and that the more we can see and understand them, the better chance we have of preventing the Earth's destruction.

That is why I have used my seminars as a means of prophecy. Again, there is no way to verify what I have found, and in time I am sure I will develop better methods for refining what those who have ventured into the far future have reported back. What I know for sure is that there is a consensus on the future from my seminar attendees, by now numbering well over two thousand, and that I am able to offer—hesitatingly, tentatively—the broad outline of a scenario I will continue to explore.

In my group progressions, as I've noted, I try to take the attendees to three stops on the journey to the future: one hundred years, five hundred years, and one thousand years from now. This is not exact. People always have the freedom to explore any realm at any time. But as a guideline, they and I find it helpful.

What have we found?

+ In one hundred years or even two hundred years the world will be pretty much the same as it is now. There have been natural and man-made calamities, tragedies, and disasters, but not on a global level. There are more toxins, more crowding, more pollution, and more global warming; there are fewer virulent diseases and better methods for growing and harvesting food, and so forth. But to paraphrase the Stephen Sondheim song, "We're still here," virtually intact.

+ After this period—it could be as near as three hundred years or as far away as six hundred—there will begin a

second Dark Ages. (In the sessions, people seem to be
foretelling ominous events closer to the earlier date.
Perhaps this is because the future is not fixed and a
blackness is advancing more quickly because of the
negative thoughts and actions of many people, though
there is still time to reverse it through our cumulative
efforts. This middle period is by far the most difficult to
pinpoint.) I don't know what caused the darkness—thus
the need for refinement—but we see a vastly diminished
population. The explanation may be a decline in fertility
rate because of poisons in the environment; already
there is ample scientific evidence that sperm motility
rates are decreasing. But viruses, poisons, asteroids,
meteors, wars, plagues, or an as yet undreamed of
calamity may also be responsible.

Some of us won't reincarnate in that time. Our consciousness may have changed enough so that we'll be
watching from another place, from another dimension.
We might not have to be here anymore. Our futures may
be more progressed individually than the future of the
planet; some of us may reincarnate in other dimensions
or worlds. In *Messages from the Masters* I wrote about a
concern that the world was moving from a one-room
schoolhouse, where first through twelfth graders were
crowded together, into two different schools, elementary
and middle. But the high school isn't here and won't be
until we stop the process of pollution, destruction, and
death. Some people have surely reached high school and
others college, but they are already in a different realm
and are arriving in larger and larger numbers. They have
reached the point where they don't have to reincarnate
on Earth anymore, and perhaps the high schoolers are
helping us from afar. Those in college are focused on
graduate school, the place where they coalesce and
become part of the One.

✦ And then the idyllic, fertile, peaceful land that Hugh
saw even before I started group progressions and that
many others have described since. Only a few attendees
have pointed out the clouds that Hugh traveled through
before reaching the bright land. Perhaps it is because we
are in those dark clouds now, and the attendees, in the
middle of them, haven't been able to recognize their
existence as Hugh did. But they all see the brightness,
they all feel the peace, and they all come back transformed. If their cumulative vision is powerful enough
and others join them in preparing for the lives to come—
rather than hating each other, killing each other, and
poisoning their environments and their souls—the ideal
realm will become manifest, and we will get to a place
on this world so like the other side that bridging them
will be easy.

Since I am mortal as well as immortal, my present concern is with
the now and the difficult time to come, for we are not forced into
that future even though our behavior seems to be limiting our options. Yet I'm optimistic. In time, I think, the people's collective
consciousness that yearns for a more peaceful and idyllic world
will achieve it. To do it, each of us must remember that our fate is
to be immortal. Alas, too many of us don't know this or in the
press of everyday events forget it.

This book, I hope, will act as a reminder.

ACKNOWLEDGMENTS

My heartfelt and enduring thanks go to Richard Marek, whose expertise and support contributed mightily to this book. He is a true friend.

The staff at Free Press has been superb throughout. Fred Hills has been invaluable since my earliest days at Simon & Schuster. He is a fantastic editor whose guidance and advice have graced my books. My deepest gratitude also goes to Carisa Hays, Elizabeth Keenan, Suzanne Donahue, Kirsa Rein, and all the others.

To my extraordinary and wonderful agent Joni Evans at the William Morris Agency, I'm eternally grateful.

And to my family, my soul mates on this life's journey and many other lifetimes as well, my supreme joy is knowing that we will always be together, to the very end of time.

ABOUT THE AUTHOR

Dr. Weiss maintains a private practice in Miami, Florida. In addition, he conducts seminars and experiential workshops nationally and internationally as well as training programs for professionals. Dr. Weiss has recorded a series of audiotapes and CDs in which he helps people discover and learn techniques of meditation, healing, deep relaxation, regression, and other visualization exercises.

For more information please contact:

The Weiss Institute
P.O. Box 560788
Miami, Florida 33256-0788

Phone: (305) 598-8151
Fax: (305) 598-4009
E-mail: in2healing@aol.com
Web site: www.brianweiss.com

PIATKUS BOOKS

If you have enjoyed reading this book, you may be interested in other titles published by Piatkus. These include:

All Piatkus titles are available from:

Piatkus Books Ltd, c/o Bookpost, PO Box 29, Douglas, Isle of Man, IM99 1BQ

Telephone (+44) 01624 677 237
Fax (+44) 01624 670 923
Email: bookshop@enterprise.net
Free Postage and Packing in the United Kingdom
Credit Cards accepted. All Cheques payable to Bookpost

Prices and availability are subject to change without prior notice. Allow 14 days for delivery.
When placing orders, please state if you do not wish to receive any additional information.